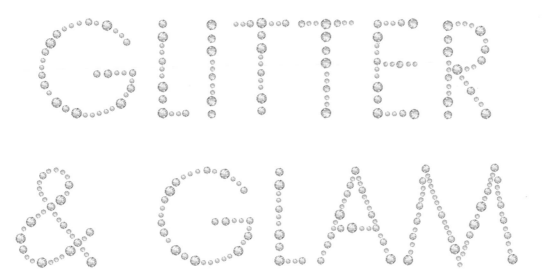

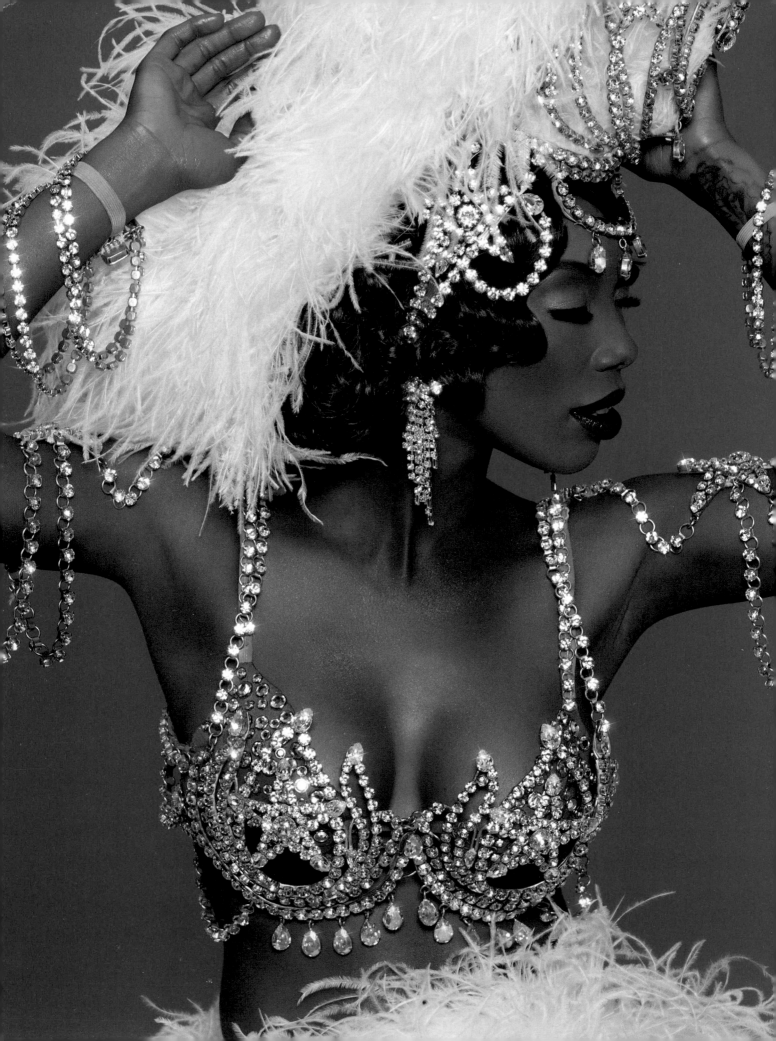

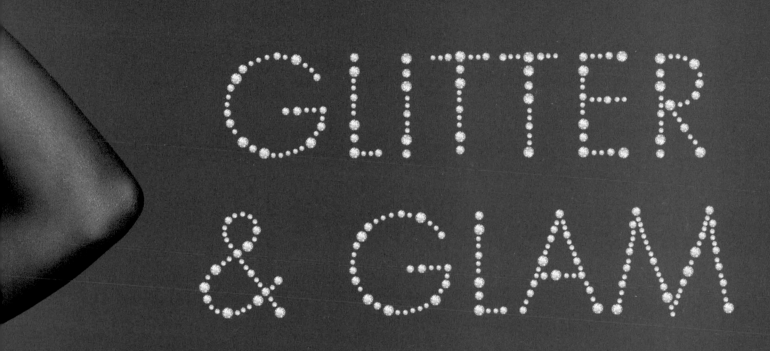

GLITTER & GLAM

dazzling makeup tips for date night,
club night, and beyond

MELANIE MILLS

A PERIGEE BOOK

A PERIGEE BOOK

Published by the Penguin Group

Penguin Group (USA)

375 Hudson Street, New York, New York 10014, USA

USA | Canada | UK | Ireland | Australia | New Zealand | India | South Africa | China

Penguin Books Ltd., Registered Offices: 80 Strand, London WC2R 0RL, England

For more information about the Penguin Group, visit penguin.com.

GLITTER & GLAM

ISBN: 978-0-399-16288-6

An application to catalog this title has been submitted to the Library of Congress.

First edition: September 2013

PRINTED IN THE UNITED STATES OF AMERICA

10 9 8 7 6 5 4 3 2 1

Photography by David Alley

Text design by Stephanie Huntwork

Most Perigee books are available at special quantity discounts for bulk purchases for sales promotions, premiums, fund-raising,
or educational use. Special books, or book excerpts, can also be created to fit specific needs. For details, write: Special.Markets@
us.penguingroup.com.

ALWAYS LEARNING   PEARSON

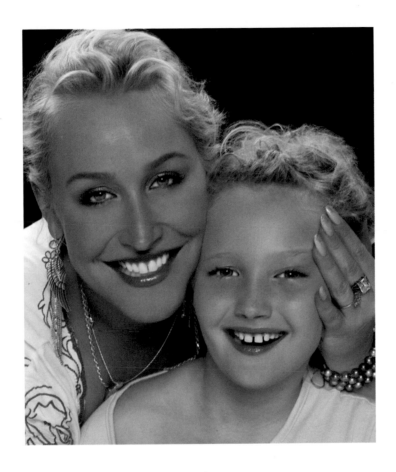

I dedicate this book to my amazing, beautiful, and smart daughter,
SOLARIS GIA BELL.
You are everything that keeps me going.
I hope to always fill your life with color and magic, as you fill mine
with sunny golden rays of love. I love you!

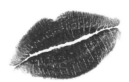

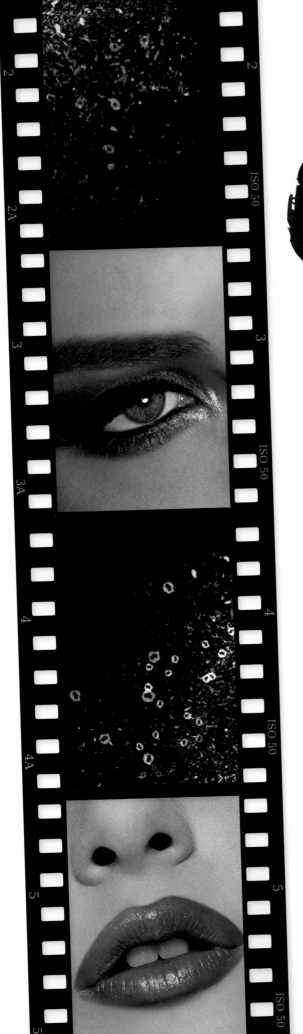

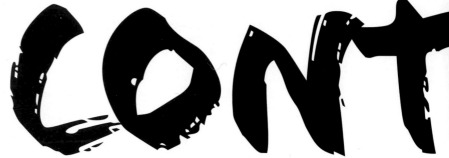

CONT

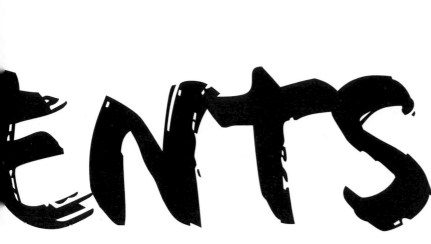

ENTS

THE LOOKS

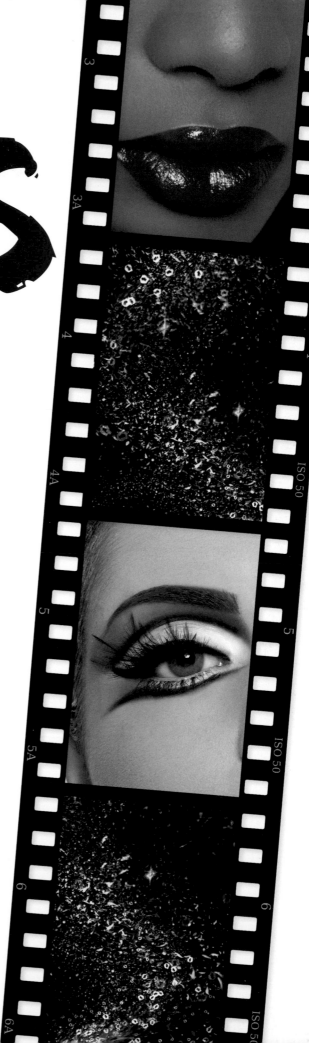

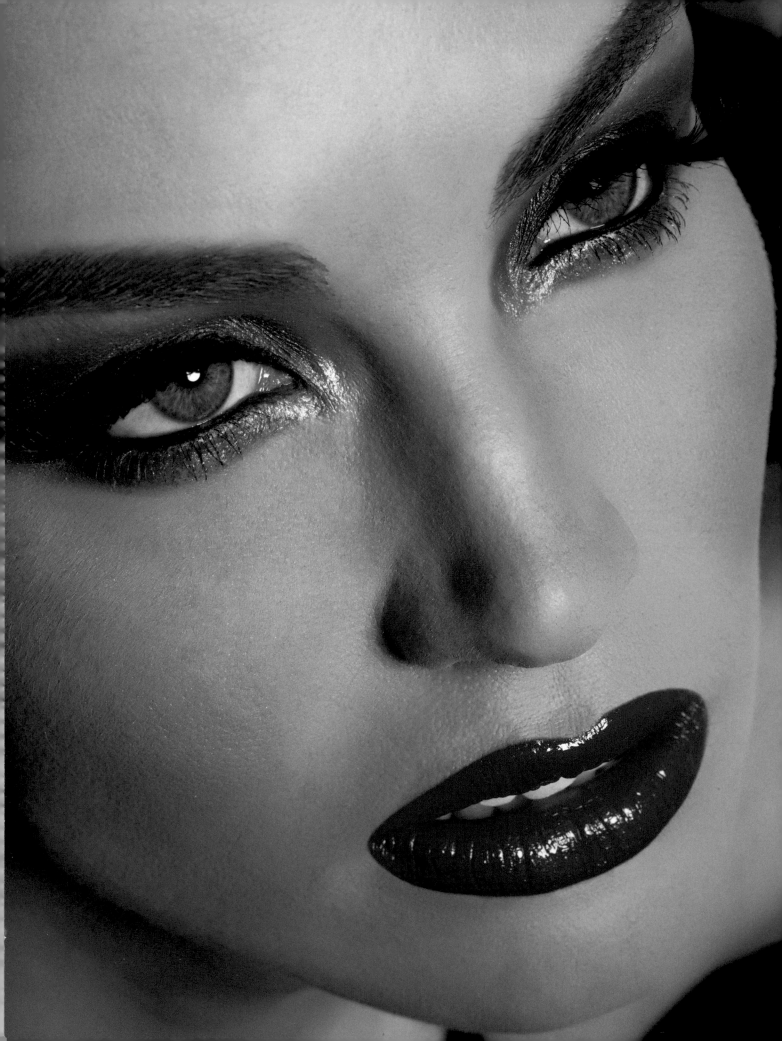

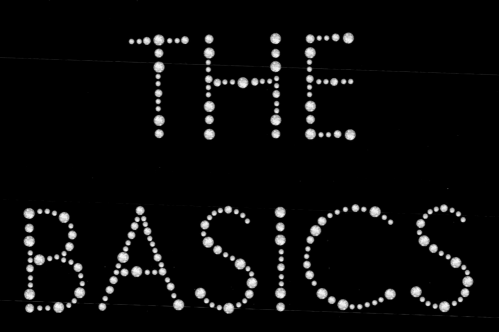

THE
BASICS

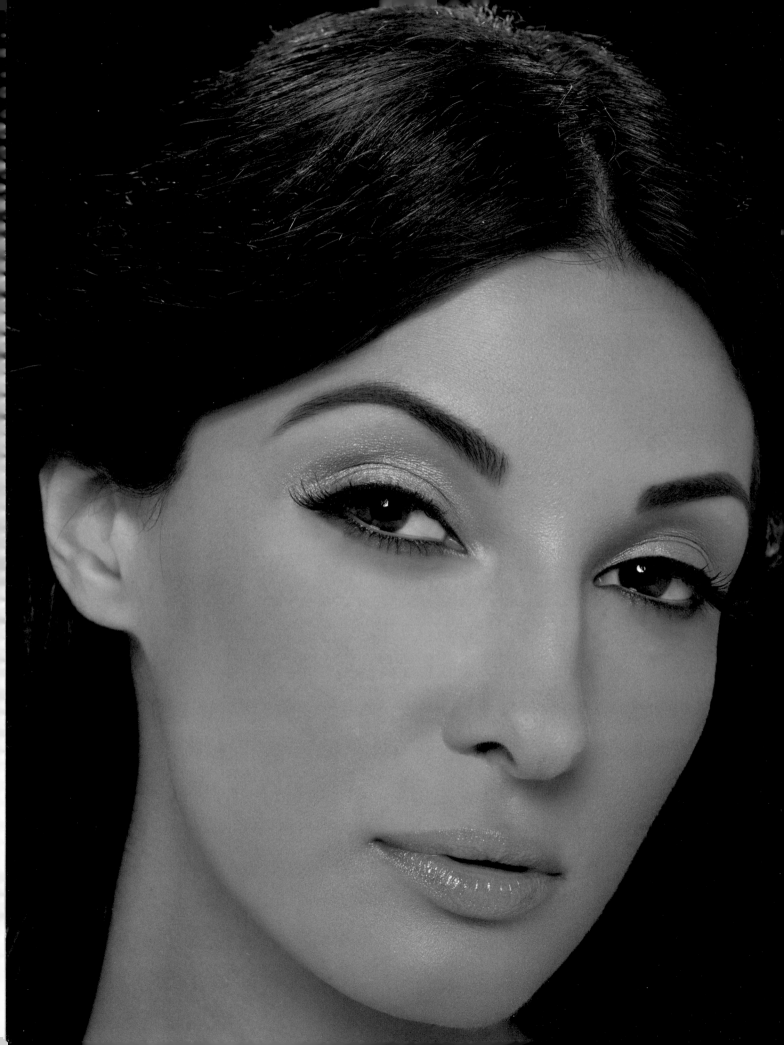

EYES

While traveling in Egypt, I will never forget descending into the depths of Queen Nefertiti's tomb. The first thing that caught my attention was a portrait of the queen herself with her beautiful eye makeup. The carbon black of the eyeliner, the royal blues of the eye shadow, the bright yellow highlights, her perfectly shaped brows, and even the gold leaf adorning her all seemed as fresh as if it had just been painted. Her eye makeup was unforgettable.

Your eyes can tell a story or make a statement without a word being spoken. The fabulous and fun thing is that you can enhance that story with makeup. You can create a mood and make yourself appear coy, fun, sexy, strong, sophisticated, or fierce. Here are my tools and tricks for perfectly stunning eyes.

EYE SHADOW PALETTES

Having many color choices of eye shadow is essential for proper eye makeup application and especially to be able to constantly change up your vibe. Make sure you have at least a couple of eye shadow palettes: one that includes great neutral shades like champagne, nude, taupe, black, and brown, and a second one with lots of bright and muted shades like purple, blue, yellow, green, and orange. Palettes make application more organized, and they are also easy to pack for travel. Some of my favorite eye shadow palettes are from Anastasia, Urban Decay, and Inglot.

CREAM SHADOWS AND LOOSE PIGMENTS

Cream eye shadow adds depth, and loose pigments add richness. A fine loose pigment blends onto your lid like nobody's business and delivers intense color. I apply cream shadow first and then lock in the color with a layer of loose pigment. You get a serious color blast that almost looks airbrushed, not to mention will last all night. (And you don't have to use them together; cream and loose pigments alone can still look fab!) When working with pigments I usually do the rest of the face makeup last, as loose pigments fall and make a mess of foundation. My favorite cream eye shadows are from Urban Decay, Make Up For Ever, Girlactik Beauty, and Cover Girl. My favorite loose pigments are from MAC, Gleam, and Make Up For Ever.

CURL

Whether applying individuals or strips, I recommend curling your natural lashes first: Gently hold the curler down on your lashes for a good ten seconds if not more unless you already have curly lashes. My favorite eyelash curler is by Tarte; it's soft and springy.

MASCARA

With strips or individual lashes, apply mascara to your real lashes before and after application, as it helps to grab the fake lash and meld to the natural ones. I use a small fan brush instead of a tube mascara wand to paint my lashes, as it's the best way to get to the root without making a mess. If using color, plastic, or fur lashes, apply mascara only before laying the lash down and not afterward. My favorite mascara is L'Oréal Voluminous Carbon Black mascara.

APPLICATION

GLUE IT

There are many eyelash adhesives, but my go-to favorites are clear and dark Duo. The dark Duo is used by most professionals; it dries black and gives the impression of a natural dark lash line. It also helps to hide the lash band. When you want that "no liner" look, find lash bands that are clear and use clear Duo. It applies white, but dries clear.

LAYERING One of my favorite techniques with individual lashes is to lay the lash in while looking down, and then look up and fill in gaps from underneath. This layering effect really ends up looking seamless and natural and makes the lashes seem very lush and full.

INDIVIDUALS/FLARES

With tweezers, grab the root of the lash and gently pull it off the box, then lightly dip the root end in the Duo. Let it air-dry for a second before setting it onto the desired point on the lash line. All sizes can be mixed together and customized. It's typical to start with minis or shorts on the inner lash line near the tear duct. As you move out toward the outer eye, you can bump up the size to short, then to medium, and then to long. It's up to the individual, the artist, and the mood you wish to create.

SINGLE STRANDS

With tweezers, grab the root of the strand and gently pull it off the box. Lightly dip the root in the glue and place it between lash strands on your lash line. Single strands are tedious to apply but great for precision placement.

STRIPS

Gently take the lash off the plastic box with your thumbs in a downward motion. Pick up and hold the lash on each side and gently bend it back and forth to loosen up the band; this helps to make it more comfortable to apply and wear. Lay the strip down on the eye without adhesive to make sure it fits. There is a natural ledge on the lash line that the strip should just fall onto. If necessary, customize the strip by cutting off a bit, or extending the lash upward off the outer lash ledge. (Instead of gluing the outer end of the lash directly onto the ledge and natural lashes, lift the end and actually glue the lash to the lid in an upward motion. This is a great trick to create a huge eye. Typically with this method you would need to fill in the gap from the false lash to the lash line with black gel liner.) Apply Duo directly onto the lash band, or use an orangewood stick for precision. Before laying down the strip on your eye, let the glue air-dry for 15 seconds to allow it to get tacky. Use either an orangewood stick, a latex triangle sponge, or the end of the Duo tube to

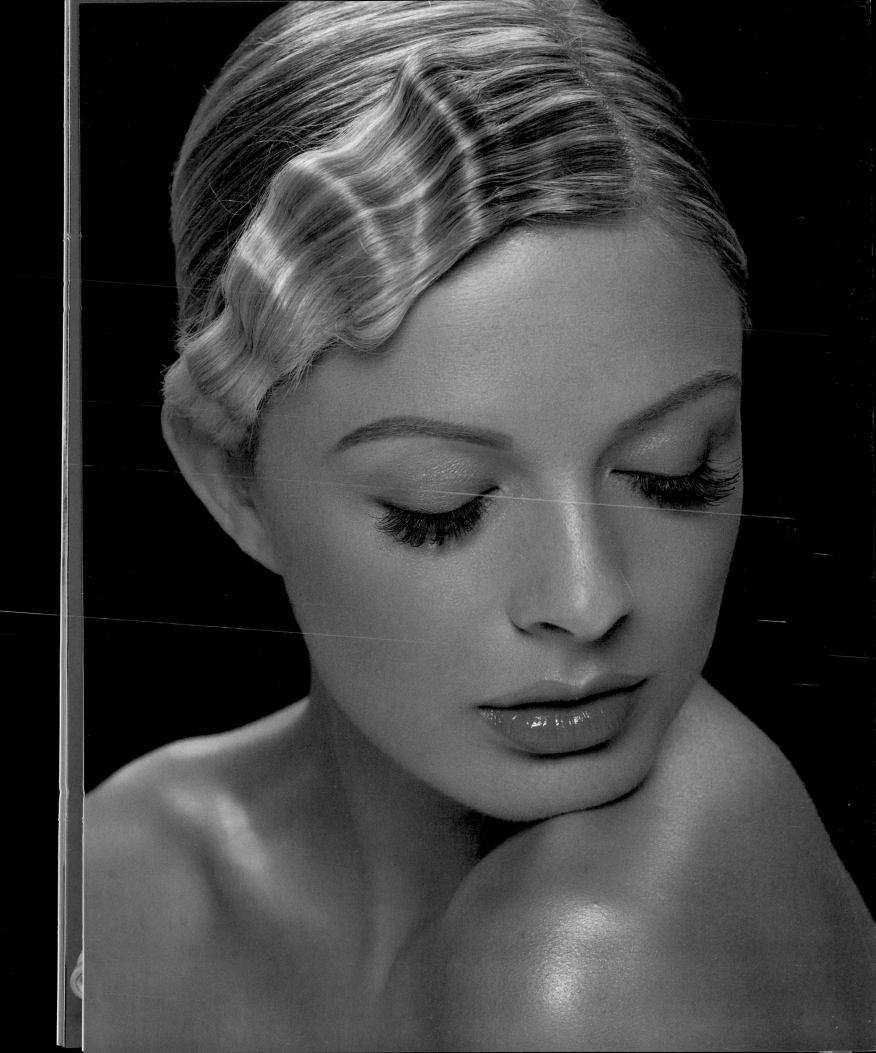

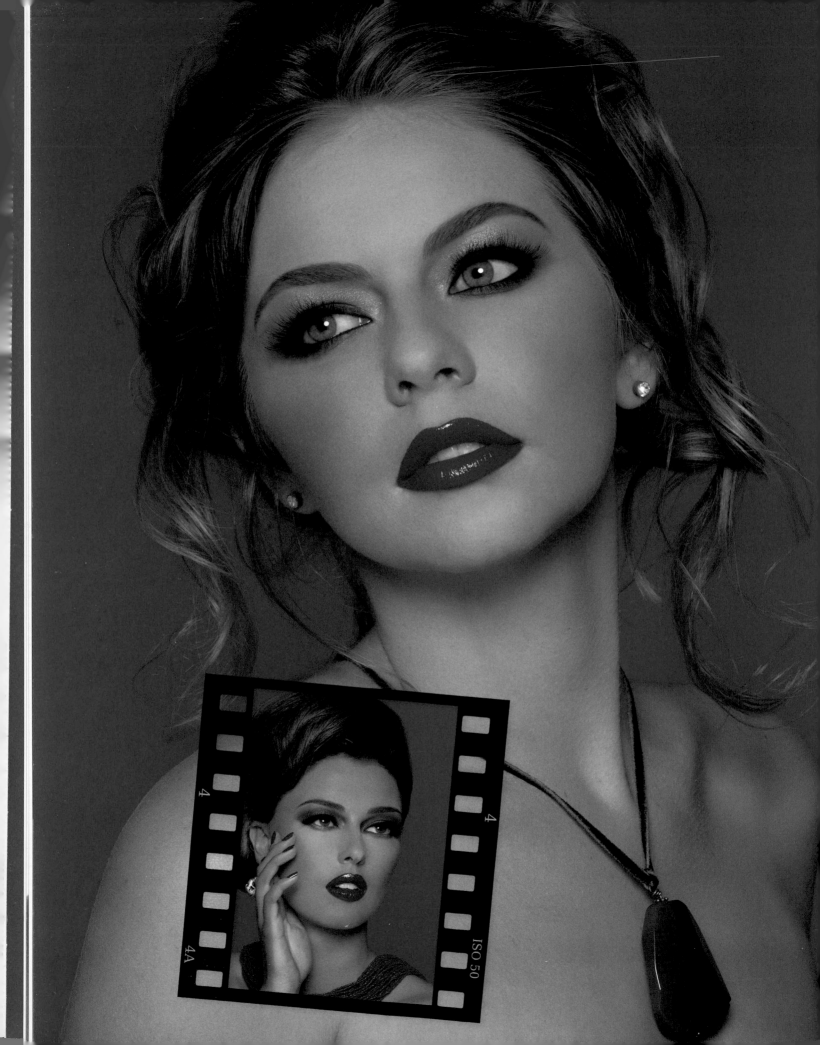

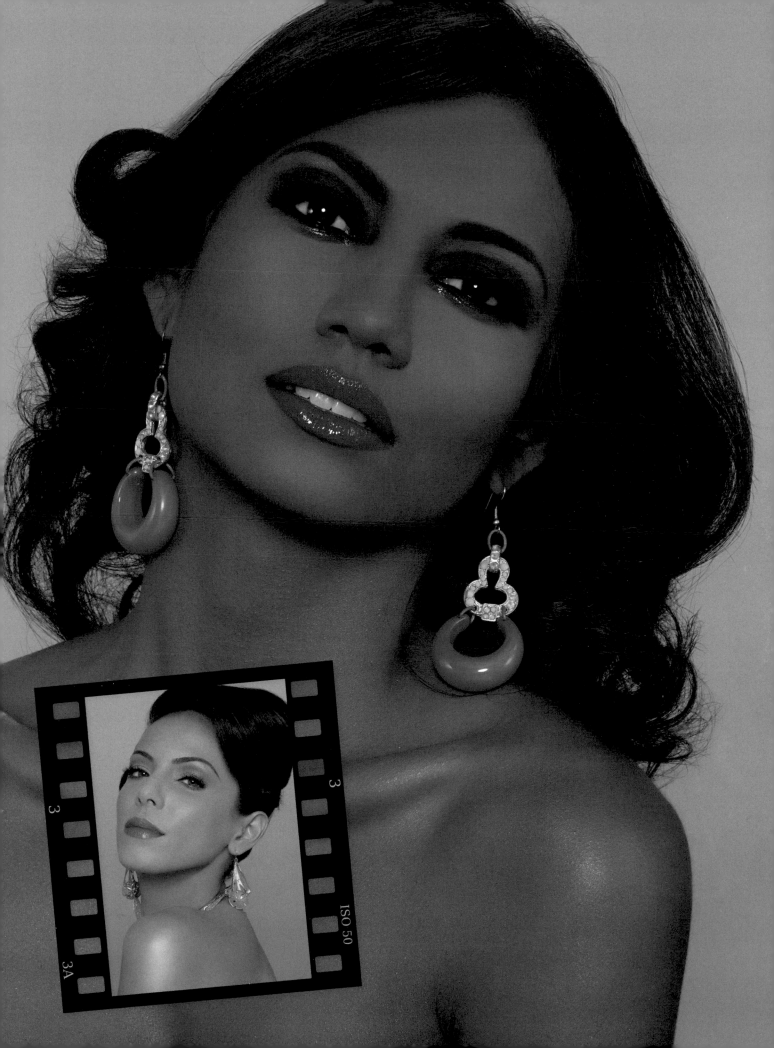

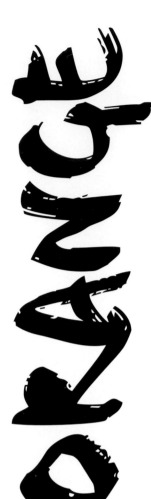

ORANGE

Orange is fall. Orange is Halloween. Orange is bold and juicy. Orange reminds me of our crazy shag carpet in the house where I grew up. Colors in the orange spectrum range from coral to soft peach. It is a great color that brightens and freshens the face. Jennette McCurdy is a talented professional, one of the hardest-working and funniest actresses I know. It's always a pleasure to work with her. Jennette is such a peach of a girl, so of course it was perfect to feature her here in orange. Sexy and fresh!

❋ Apply foundation to all of the face, neck, and eyes.

❋ Contour from under the cheekbones and jawline and down the sides of the nose with gray/taupe cream contour color.

❋ Apply a bright peach cream blush to the cheekbones.

❋ Blend this all in with foundation brushes and a Beautyblender.

❋ Lightly powder the face with translucent powder.

❋ Fill in the brows (lightly, so it looks natural) with clear wax and taupe eyebrow shadow; using an angled eyebrow brush, brush out the beginnings of the brow upward.

❋ Using an eye shadow brush, apply bone-colored cream eye shadow all over the eye up under the brow.

❋ With an eye shadow brush, apply rose gold shimmery loose powder onto the lid.

❋ Apply bright orange loose pigment to the outer corner of the eye, blending back into the crease.

❋ Line the inner upper and lower waterlines with a brown gel liner.

❋ Tightly line the top lash line, and then buff it out with a small blunt eye shadow brush to soften.

❋ Using a small blunt eye shadow brush, blend over the liner at the lash line with a shimmery soft brown eye shadow; apply it under all of the eye and up around the outer corner of the eye.

❋ Line the upper lash line again with a small pointy eyeliner brush. I know we already did this, but all of these actions create depth, and this final sweep creates precision.

❋ Curl the lashes and apply mascara.

❋ Apply individual flare lashes in short, medium, and long, in layers, using dark Duo.

❋ Apply mascara again.

❋ Dust rose gold shimmery loose powder onto the cheeks using a fluffy blush brush.

❋ Line and fill in the lips with a tangerine lip pencil.

❋ Apply a peach lip gloss on top.

❋ Use rose gold body makeup all over the body.

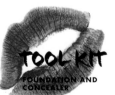

TOOL KIT

FOUNDATION AND CONCEALER

GRAY/TAUPE CREAM CONTOUR COLOR

BRIGHT PEACH CREAM BLUSH

TRANSLUCENT POWDER

CLEAR WAX AND TAUPE EYEBROW SHADOW

BONE-COLORED CREAM EYE SHADOW

ROSE GOLD SHIMMERY LOOSE POWDER

BRIGHT ORANGE LOOSE PIGMENT

BROWN GEL LINER

SHIMMERY SOFT BROWN EYE SHADOW

BLACK MASCARA

INDIVIDUAL FLARE LASHES IN SHORT, MEDIUM, AND LONG

DARK DUO

TANGERINE LIP PENCIL

PEACH LIP GLOSS

ROSE GOLD BODY MAKEUP

FOUNDATION BRUSHES

BEAUTYBLENDER

POWDER BRUSH

ANGLED EYEBROW BRUSH

EYEBROW COMB

EYE SHADOW BRUSHES

SMALL POINTY EYELINER BRUSH

EYELASH CURLER

SMALL FAN BRUSH

TWEEZERS

FLUFFY BLUSH BRUSH

LIP BRUSH

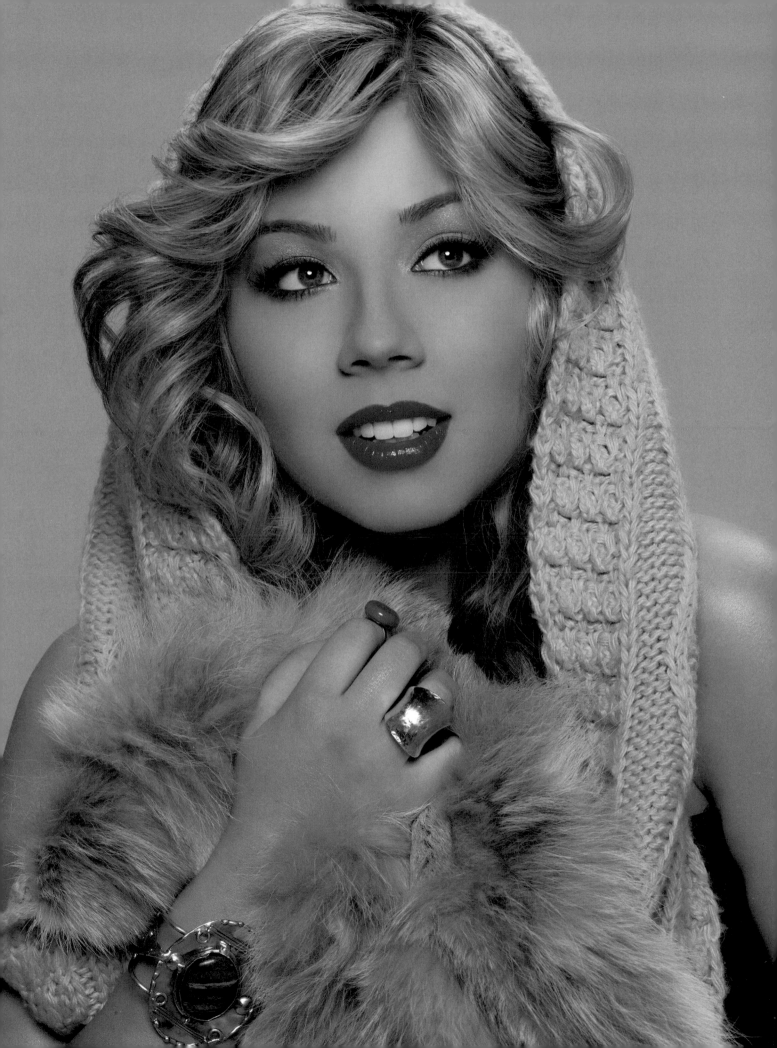

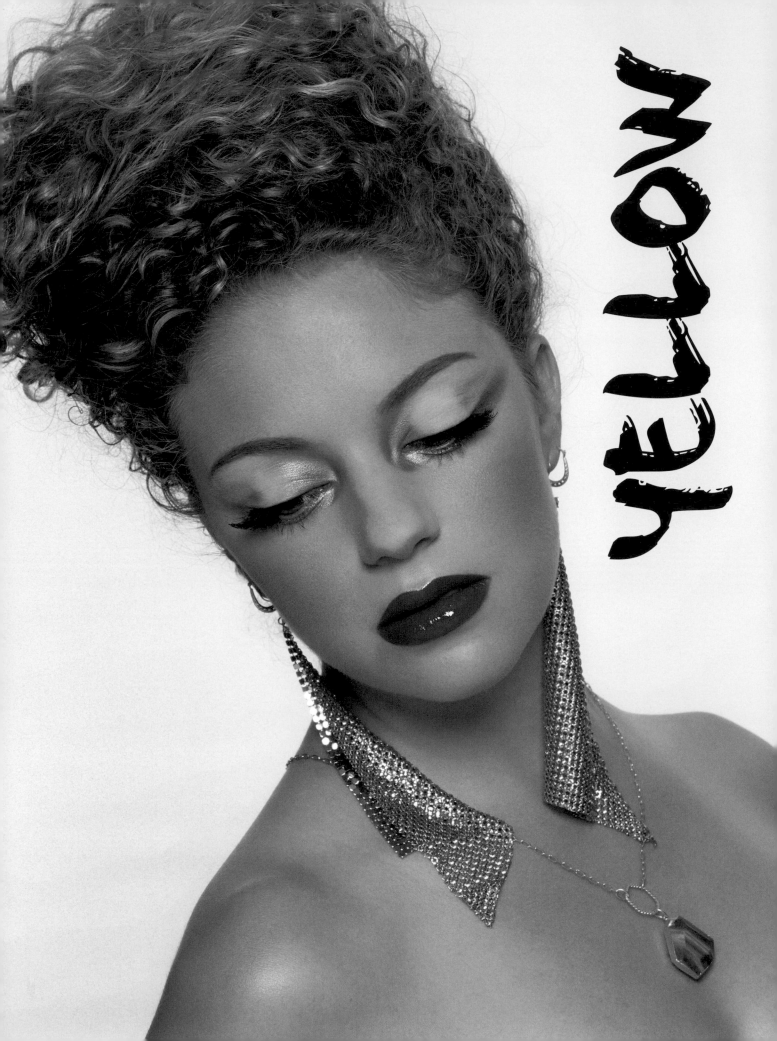

YELLOW

Yellow is happy. Yellow is friendship. Yellow is sunshine. Yellow reminds me of my kitchen on a sunny summer morning. I love mixing yellows and golds into makeup; it's a great transition color and can make a sexy bold statement on its own. Shelby is perfect! Combining gold and yellow, she becomes even more radiant. Get your glam disco on!

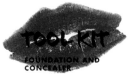

* Apply foundation all over the eyes, up onto the forehead, and into the hairline.

* With a medium taupe eyebrow pencil, draw in the eyebrow shape naturally.

* Use a medium taupe eyebrow shadow and an angled eyebrow brush to extend the end of the brow.

* With an eye shadow brush, apply a soft pale yellow gold shimmery eye shadow all over the eyelids.

* With an eye shadow brush, apply metallic gold loose pigment in a circular motion to the inner eye all the way up to the brow, then brush the gold around the tear duct and all the way below the eye; flare out under the outer eye toward the temple to a dramatic point.

* Using a thin crease eye shadow brush, apply matte white eye shadow to the outer corner of the eye on top of the gold; flare out off the eye toward the temple.

* Apply a matte, very pigmented, bright yellow eye shadow to the middle of the eyelid from the lash line all the way up to the brow. Extend the color under the eyebrow, flaring out on top of the white flare; make sure to get a lot of the color onto the brush, layering the color a few times for that extra pop factor.

* Line the upper lash line with brown gel liner using a small pointy eyeliner brush; keep the line tight and just to the end of the eye, no flare out.

* Line the inner lower waterline with a white eyeliner pencil.

* Curl the lashes and apply mascara.

* Layer lots of individual flare lashes in short, medium, and long with dark Duo.

* Apply mascara again.

* Go over the upper gel eyeliner one more time for extra freshness.

* Apply foundation to the rest of the face, neck, and ears.

* Contour down the sides of the nose, under the cheekbones, and along the jawline with a gray/taupe cream color.

* Apply a sheer red cream blush to the cheeks.

* Blend this all in with foundation brushes and a Beautyblender.

* Lightly powder the face with translucent powder.

* Using a blush brush, apply a shimmery coral blush to the apples of the cheeks; blend up toward the outer eye.

* Lightly dust on a sheer reddish bronze gold loose powder to the upper cheekbones, temples, jaw, and neck with a fluffy blush brush, to give that sun-kissed look.

* Line and fill in the lips with a red lip pencil.

* Top off the lips with a bright orange red lip gloss.

TOOL KIT

FOUNDATION AND CONCEALER

MEDIUM TAUPE EYEBROW PENCIL

MEDIUM TAUPE EYEBROW SHADOW

SOFT PALE YELLOW GOLD SHIMMERY EYE SHADOW

METALLIC GOLD LOOSE PIGMENT

MATTE WHITE EYE SHADOW

MATTE, VERY PIGMENTED, BRIGHT YELLOW EYE SHADOW

BROWN GEL LINER

WHITE EYELINER PENCIL

BLACK MASCARA

INDIVIDUAL FLARE LASHES IN SHORT, MEDIUM, AND LONG

DARK DUO

GRAY/TAUPE CREAM CONTOUR COLOR

SHEER RED CREAM BLUSH

SHIMMERY CORAL BLUSH

SHEER REDDISH BRONZE GOLD LOOSE POWDER

RED LIP PENCIL

BRIGHT ORANGE RED LIP GLOSS

FOUNDATION BRUSHES

BEAUTYBLENDER

ANGLED EYEBROW BRUSH

EYE SHADOW BRUSHES

SMALL POINTY EYELINER BRUSH

EYELASH CURLER

SMALL FAN BRUSH

TWEEZERS

POWDER BRUSH

BLUSH BRUSHES

LIP BRUSH

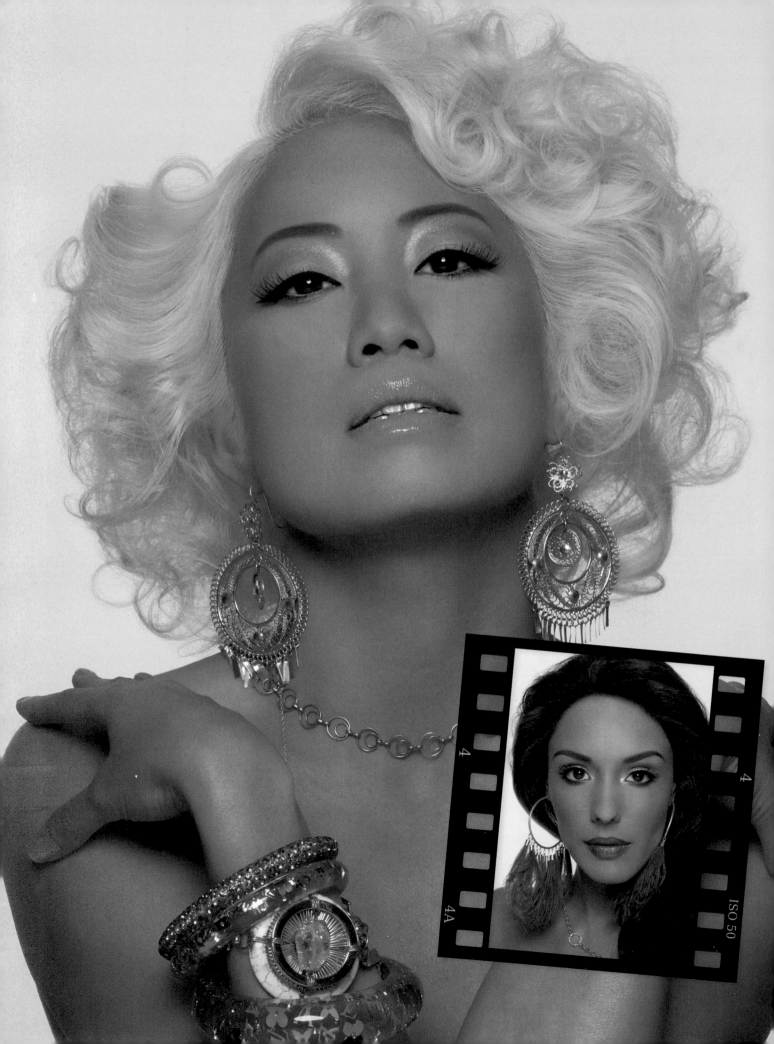

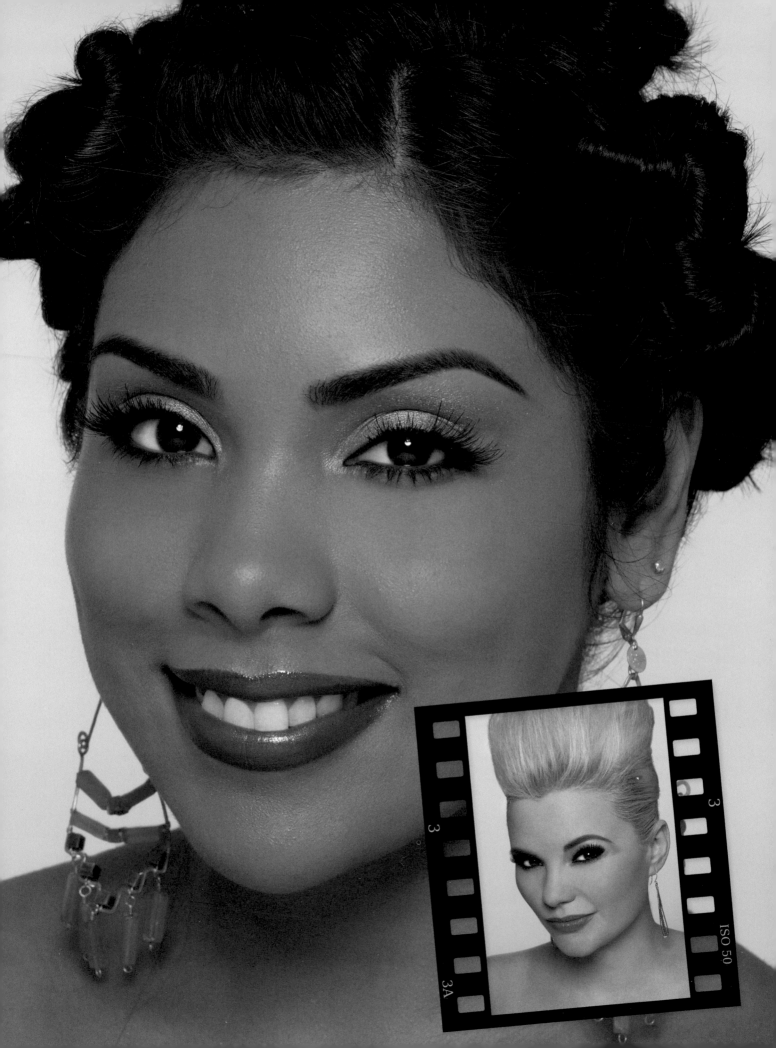

Green is far from just a buzzword that describes an eco movement. Green is nature. Green is free, and it's fun! I met Jessica while working on an NBC show called *The Taste*. This is a sexy, glamorous, fun look, sure to turn heads when out on the town.

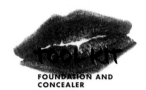

TOOL KIT

FOUNDATION AND CONCEALER

MEDIUM BROWN EYEBROW PENCIL

CLEAR WAX AND LIGHT BROWN EYEBROW SHADOW

METALLIC HUNTER GREEN CREAM EYE SHADOW

METALLIC HUNTER GREEN LOOSE PIGMENT

YELLOW OLIVE GREEN LOOSE PIGMENT

BLACK SHIMMERY EYE SHADOW

BLACK GEL LINER

YELLOW OLIVE GREEN GLITTER

EMERALD GREEN GLITTER

DARK AND CLEAR DUO

WATER

BLACK MASCARA

ONE SET WISPIES STRIP LASHES

1 SET SEPARATED POINTY DRAMATIC FIERCE STRIP LASHES

ROSE GOLD MAKEUP

BRIGHT BEIGE/PINK CREAM BLUSH

GRAY/TAUPE CREAM CONTOUR COLOR

TRANSLUCENT POWDER

ROSE GOLD LOOSE POWDER

GLOSSY LIP BALM

FOUNDATION BRUSHES

BEAUTYBLENDER

ANGLED EYEBROW BRUSH

EYE SHADOW BRUSHES

EYELINER BRUSH

EYELASH CURLER

ROUNDED Q-TIPS

CERAMIC BOWL

TISSUE

EYELASH COMB

SCOTCH TAPE

SMALL FAN BRUSH

ORANGEWOOD STICK

POWDER BRUSH

BLUSH BRUSH

LIP BRUSH

* Apply foundation; brush over the eyes and forehead and into the hairline.

* Using a medium brown eyebrow pencil, draw in the brow well above the normal arch and extend it out toward the temple.

* Use clear wax and a light brown eyebrow shadow to fill in on top of the eyebrow pencil.

* With a small eye shadow brush, apply metallic hunter green cream eye shadow over the lid to the crease, extending the color out to the end of the brow. Apply the same color under the eye around the tear duct, flaring out and up in a circular motion, connecting the color.

* Using the same hunter green color in a loose pigment, go over the cream with an eye shadow brush to intensify the color and to lock in the cream.

* With a yellow olive green loose pigment, highlight the upper inner eye and around the tear duct by blending in circular motions with a small eye shadow brush.

* With a black shimmery eye shadow and a thin eye shadow brush, lightly apply a sideways *V* shape from the middle crease to the outer eye and then down under the outer corner. Use a clean eye shadow brush to blend out.

* Line the upper and lower inner waterlines with a black gel liner. Also line the upper lash line from the tear duct to the outer eye, finishing with a tight swoop.

* Dip a rounded Q-tip into a thick clear Duo wash, lightly close the eyes, and tap (lightly so as not to remove the eye shadow) onto the lid anywhere you want the glitter applied. Dip the same Q-tip into the glitter and tap the glitter onto the wash quickly and evenly. Keep repeating these steps until satisfied, switching out Q-tips often.

* For this look, use a yellow olive green glitter for the inner eye and an emerald green glitter for the outer eye.

* Once done with the glitter, keep the eyes still lightly closed, then bend forward and use a short clean eye shadow brush to dust off unwanted glitter. Then, with an eyelash comb, brush out the eyelashes.

* Remove the tissue and brush the glitter off the face, using Scotch tape to remove the last bits. Slowly open the eyes.

* Apply mascara with a small fan brush.

* Apply Wispies strip lashes followed by a set of large spiky vampy lashes on top, using dark Duo. Apply mascara again.

* Apply foundation to the rest of the face, neck, and ears.

* Mix a rose gold makeup into the foundation and, with a Beautyblender, apply the mix from the upper cheek to the jaw and onto the neck.

* Apply a bright beige/pink cream blush to the cheeks.

* Contour the jaw with a gray/taupe cream contour color.

* Blend this all in with foundation brushes and a Beautyblender.

* Powder with translucent powder all over the face and neck.

* With a blush brush, apply rose gold loose powder to the cheeks up to the temple.

* Apply a glossy lip balm to the lips.

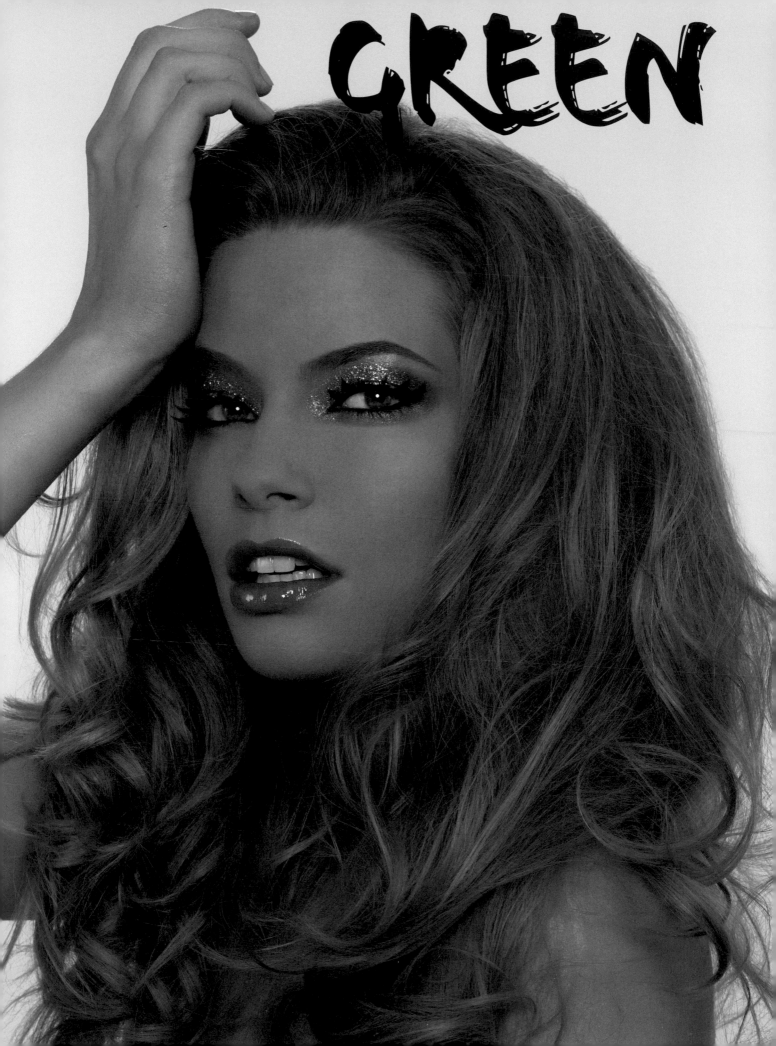

GREEN

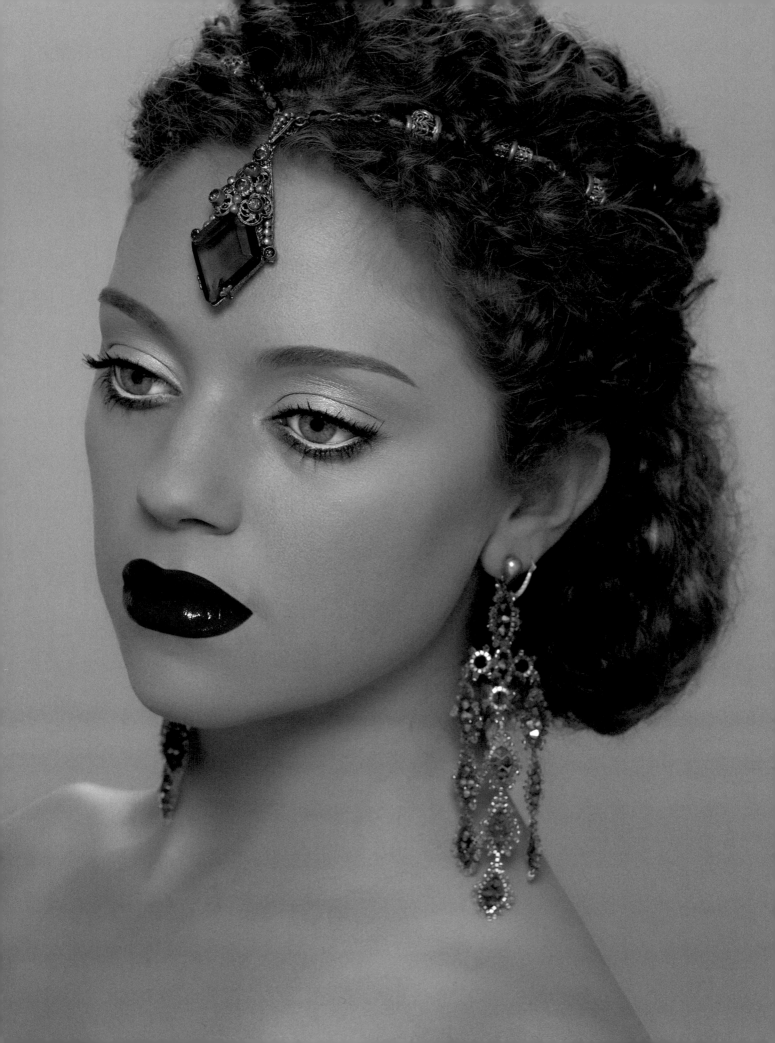

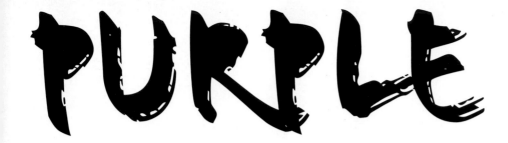

PURPLE

Purple is royal. Purple is rich. Purple is relaxing. Purple is exotic. Shelby is another great find from Nickelodeon's *Victorious*. She is a stunning beauty and so nice. This look depicted her holding court in Old Spain. It's bold, yet exquisite, and quite simple to achieve. The lips make this look even bolder, which is ideal for a romantic dinner or night out.

* Apply foundation to the whole face, eyes, neck, and ears. Do not contour; the face should be very soft.

* Apply a pale pink cream blush to the apples of the cheeks.

* Blend this all in with foundation brushes and a Beautyblender.

* Powder the face with translucent powder and a powder puff.

* Use clear wax and a taupe eyebrow shadow with an angled eyebrow brush to fill in naturally.

* With an eye shadow brush, apply a very light yet shimmery lavender eye shadow to the lid up to the crease and just extend to the outer eye ever so slightly.

* Using a short eye shadow brush, apply a bright purple eye shadow just under the eye.

* With a small thin crease brush, apply the same shadow very lightly and gently to crease and blend out, to make just a trace of a contour.

* Clean up under the brow with a small foundation brush and a bit of foundation.

* Line the inner lower waterline with a white eyeliner pencil. Go back and forth a few times and take the color around the inner tear duct.

* Curl the lashes and apply mascara.

* Lightly brush an iridescent loose powder all under the eye, then out in an upward motion to add a bit of highlight.

* Apply soft peach blush to the upper cheekbones with a fluffy blush brush.

* With a dark eggplant lip pencil, line the lips dramatically, then fill all the way.

* Finish off with a bright cranberry lipstick.

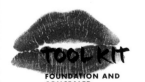

TOOLKIT

FOUNDATION AND CONCEALER

PALE PINK CREAM BLUSH

TRANSLUCENT POWDER

CLEAR WAX AND TAUPE EYEBROW SHADOW

PALE SHIMMERY LAVENDER EYE SHADOW

BRIGHT PURPLE EYE SHADOW

WHITE EYELINER PENCIL

BLACK MASCARA

IRIDESCENT LOOSE POWDER

SOFT PEACH BLUSH

DARK EGGPLANT LIP PENCIL

BRIGHT CRANBERRY LIPSTICK

FOUNDATION BRUSHES

BEAUTYBLENDER

POWDER PUFF

ANGLED EYEBROW BRUSH

EYE SHADOW BRUSHES

EYELINER BRUSHES

EYELASH CURLER

SMALL FAN BRUSH

SMALL POWDER BRUSH

BLUSH BRUSH

LIP BRUSH

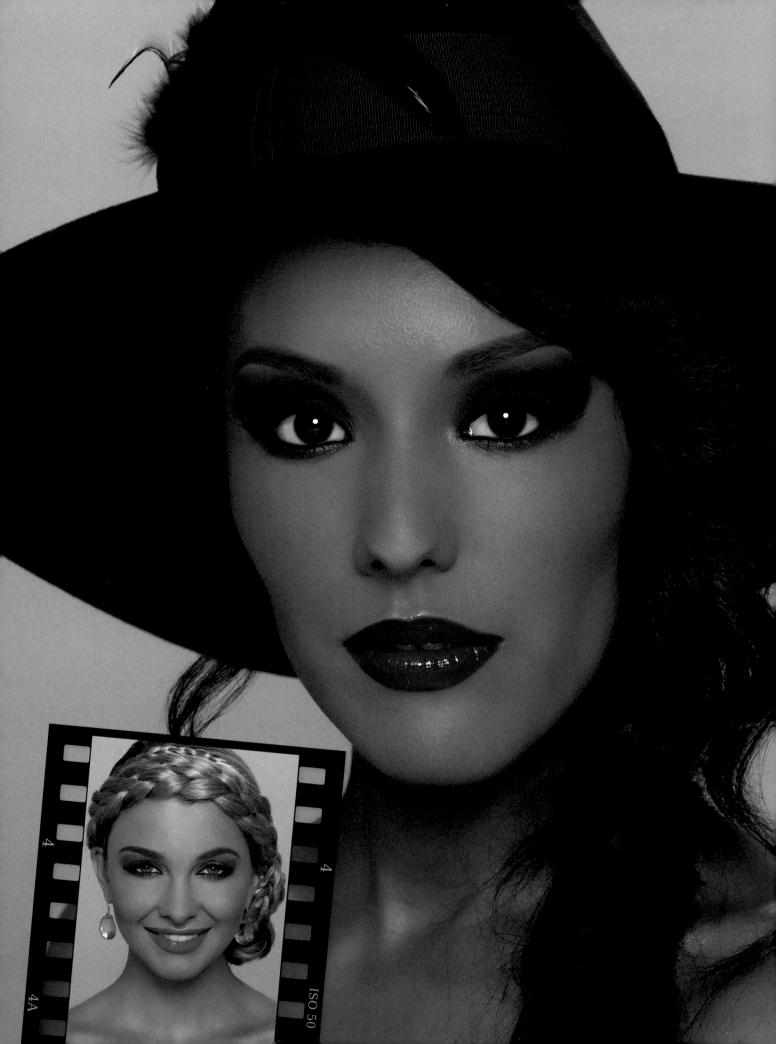

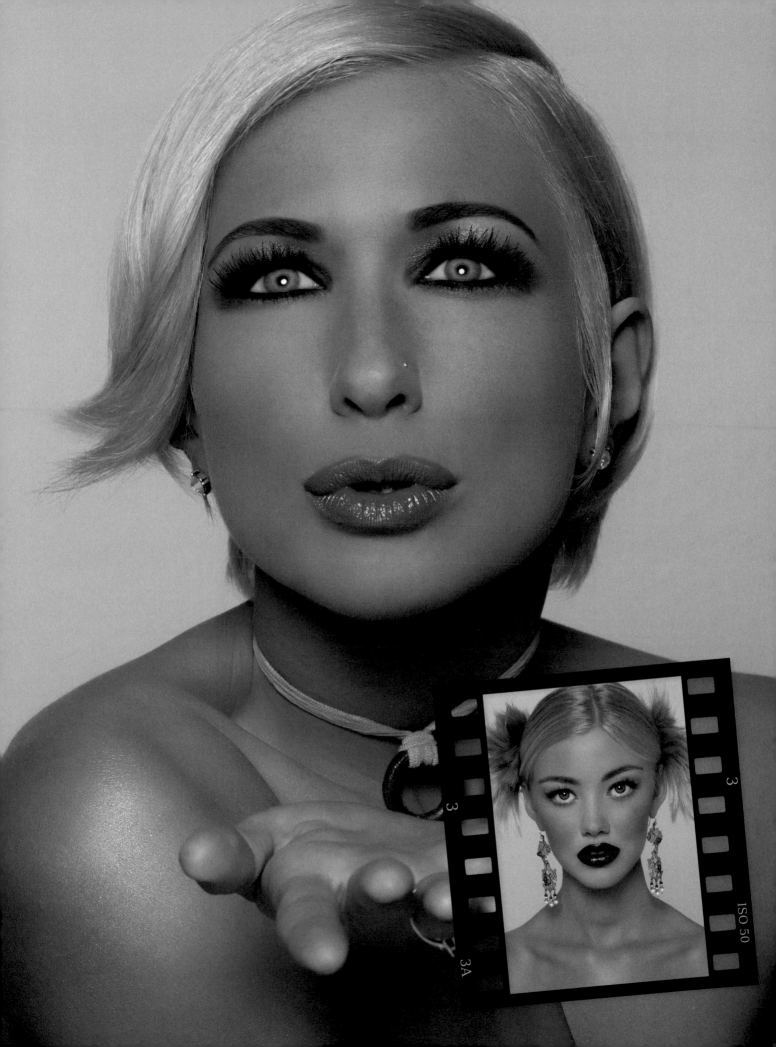

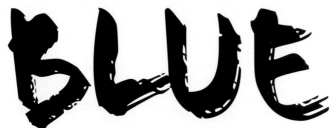

BLUE

Blue is timeless. Blue oceans and skies are infinite. Blue is peaceful, yet it can also be electric! Blue is one of my favorite colors and can be worn by almost anybody. With Denise, a friend of my photographer, David Alley, I wanted to use a combination of a soft, soothing blue and an electric blue. This is a look that is intensely, alluringly cool!

* Apply foundation all over the eyes and up to the forehead.

* Brush out the eyebrows, then fill in with clear wax and dark brown eyebrow shadow using an angled eyebrow brush.

* With a regular eye shadow brush, apply baby blue sparkly eye shadow; go over the whole lid up to the crease, extending out just a touch, blending the outside corner in a circular motion.

* With a thin eye shadow brush, apply a brighter, bolder blue eye shadow to the crease, again extending out a touch; blend the outer eye in a circular motion for a rounded shape.

* With a royal bright blue cream eye shadow and a thick eyeliner brush, line all the way under the eye to the outer corner, extending slightly onto the upper lid. With a smaller pointy eyeliner brush, draw a cat line on the upper lash line, connecting the outer under and upper corners. Also line all the way around the tear duct.

* With a small blunt eye shadow brush, apply a bright shimmery topaz blue loose pigment over the cream all the way around the eye to intensify the color and lock in the cream.

* For the inner upper and lower waterlines, use a navy blue gel liner with a soft pointy eyeliner brush to line the inner tear duct as well.

* Curl the lashes and apply mascara.

* Lay in several black individual flare lashes in short, medium, and long with dark Duo.

* Apply mascara again.

* Clean up under the eyes with makeup remover.

* Apply foundation to the rest of the face, neck, and ears and under the brow bone.

* Contour down the outside of the nose, under the cheekbones, and on the jawline with a brown cream contour color.

* Apply a burnt rose cream blush.

* Blend this all in with foundation brushes and a Beautyblender.

* Lightly powder the whole face with peach loose powder.

* Apply shimmery rose gold loose powder to the cheeks with a fluffy blush brush.

* Line and fill in the lips with a nude or spice pencil.

* Top off the lips with a caramel-colored lip gloss.

* Apply rose gold body makeup all over the body.

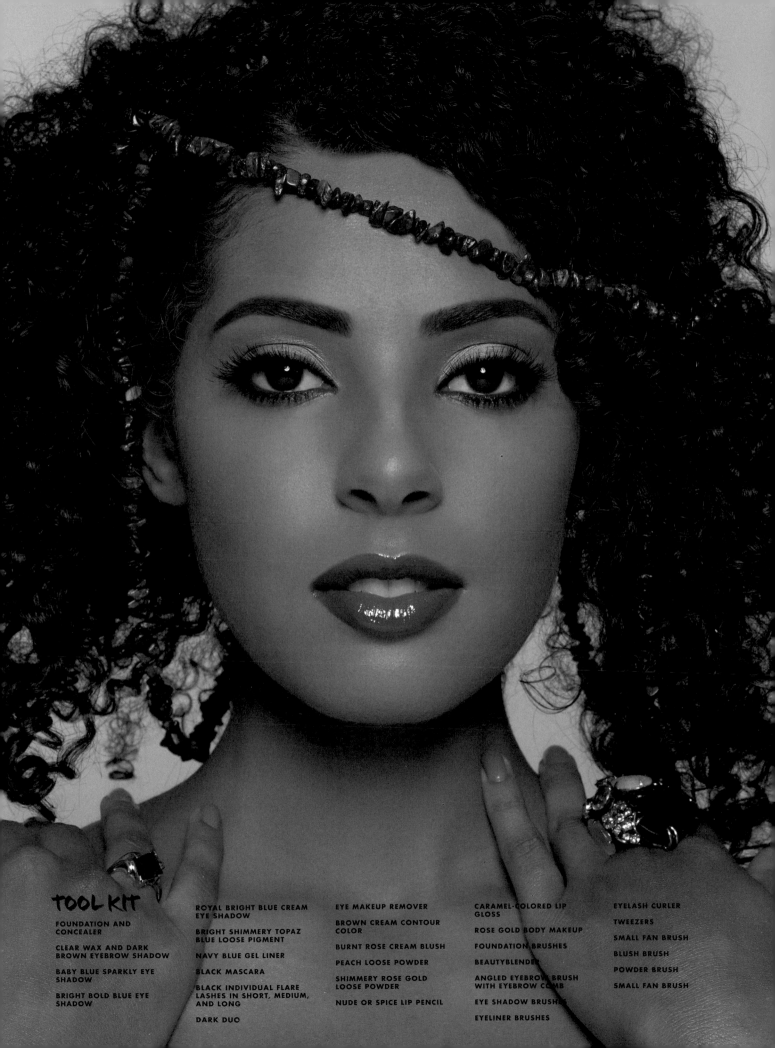

TOOL KIT

FOUNDATION AND
CONCEALER

CLEAR WAX AND DARK
BROWN EYEBROW SHADOW

BABY BLUE SPARKLY EYE
SHADOW

BRIGHT BOLD BLUE EYE
SHADOW

ROYAL BRIGHT BLUE CREAM
EYE SHADOW

BRIGHT SHIMMERY TOPAZ
BLUE LOOSE PIGMENT

NAVY BLUE GEL LINER

BLACK MASCARA

BLACK INDIVIDUAL FLARE
LASHES IN SHORT, MEDIUM,
AND LONG

DARK DUO

EYE MAKEUP REMOVER

BROWN CREAM CONTOUR
COLOR

BURNT ROSE CREAM BLUSH

PEACH LOOSE POWDER

SHIMMERY ROSE GOLD
LOOSE POWDER

NUDE OR SPICE LIP PENCIL

CARAMEL-COLORED LIP
GLOSS

ROSE GOLD BODY MAKEUP

FOUNDATION BRUSHES

BEAUTYBLENDER

ANGLED EYEBROW BRUSH
WITH EYEBROW COMB

EYE SHADOW BRUSHES

EYELINER BRUSHES

EYELASH CURLER

TWEEZERS

SMALL FAN BRUSH

BLUSH BRUSH

POWDER BRUSH

SMALL FAN BRUSH

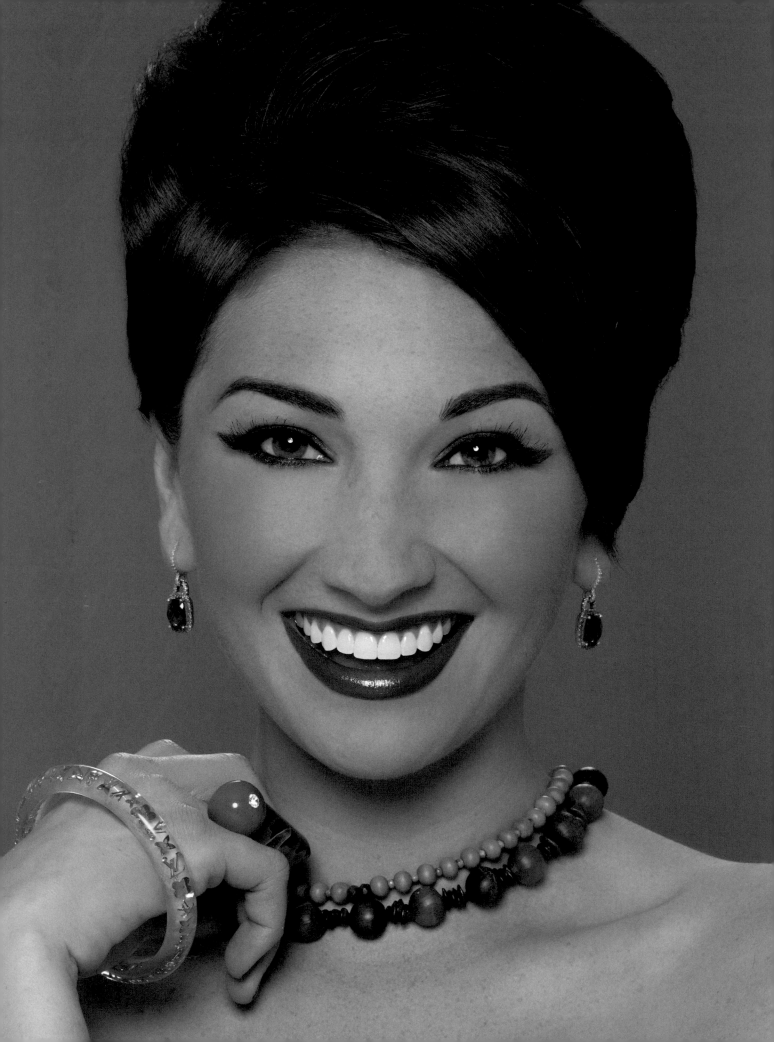

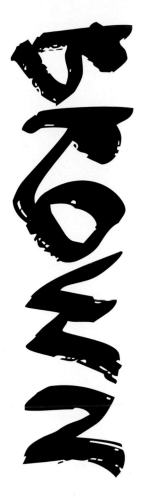

Brown is cozy. Brown is earthy. Brown is a beautiful Tahitian tan. Brown is warm. Brown is a key color in most makeup palettes, from rich chocolates to taupes to rust and copper. I did a young, sweet ode to *Breakfast at Tiffany's*. Maddie's sweet freckles and hair inspired this classic look. I added a twist to celebrate the many shades of brown.

* Apply foundation to the whole face, eyes, neck, and ears.

* Apply a nude rose-colored cream blush to the apples of the cheeks and then blend up toward the ears.

* Blend this all in with foundation brushes and a Beautyblender.

* Lightly dust the face with translucent powder.

* Sculpt the eyebrows by drawing them in first with a thin brown eyebrow pencil and then softening and extending them with an angled eyebrow brush and a dark brown eyebrow shadow.

* With an eye shadow brush, apply a matte warm apricot eye shadow lightly over the lid and up to the crease, and then blend out the edges with a clean eye shadow brush.

* Use a brown gel liner to draw a nice elegant cat line, extending up and out, thicker at the end, and then back down, connecting under the outer eye. Also line the inner upper and lower waterlines.

* With a copper brown eye shadow and an eyeliner brush, go over the gel liner.

* Curl the lashes and apply mascara.

* Apply individual flare lashes in short, medium, and long all over the lash line with clear Duo.

* Apply mascara again.

* Add a peachy bronze blush with a blush brush over the cheeks.

* Use a brown lip pencil to fill in the lips and draw a beautiful lip line.

* Apply a bronze brown sparkly lipstick on top of the lips with a lip brush.

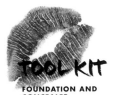

TOOL KIT

FOUNDATION AND CONCEALER	**DARK BROWN EYEBROW SHADOW**	**INDIVIDUAL FLARE LASHES IN SHORT, MEDIUM, AND LONG**	**FOUNDATION BRUSHES**	**EYELASH CURLER**
NUDE ROSE-COLORED CREAM BLUSH	**MATTE WARM APRICOT EYE SHADOW**	**CLEAR DUO**	**BEAUTYBLENDER**	**TWEEZERS**
TRANSLUCENT POWDER	**BROWN GEL LINER**	**PEACHY BRONZE BLUSH**	**BLUSH BRUSH**	**SMALL FAN BRUSH**
THIN BROWN EYEBROW PENCIL	**COPPER BROWN EYE SHADOW**	**BROWN LIP PENCIL**	**POWDER BRUSH**	**LIP BRUSH**
	LIGHT BLACK MASCARA	**BRONZE BROWN SPARKLY LIPSTICK**	**ANGLED EYEBROW BRUSH**	
			EYE SHADOW BRUSHES	
			EYELINER BRUSHES	

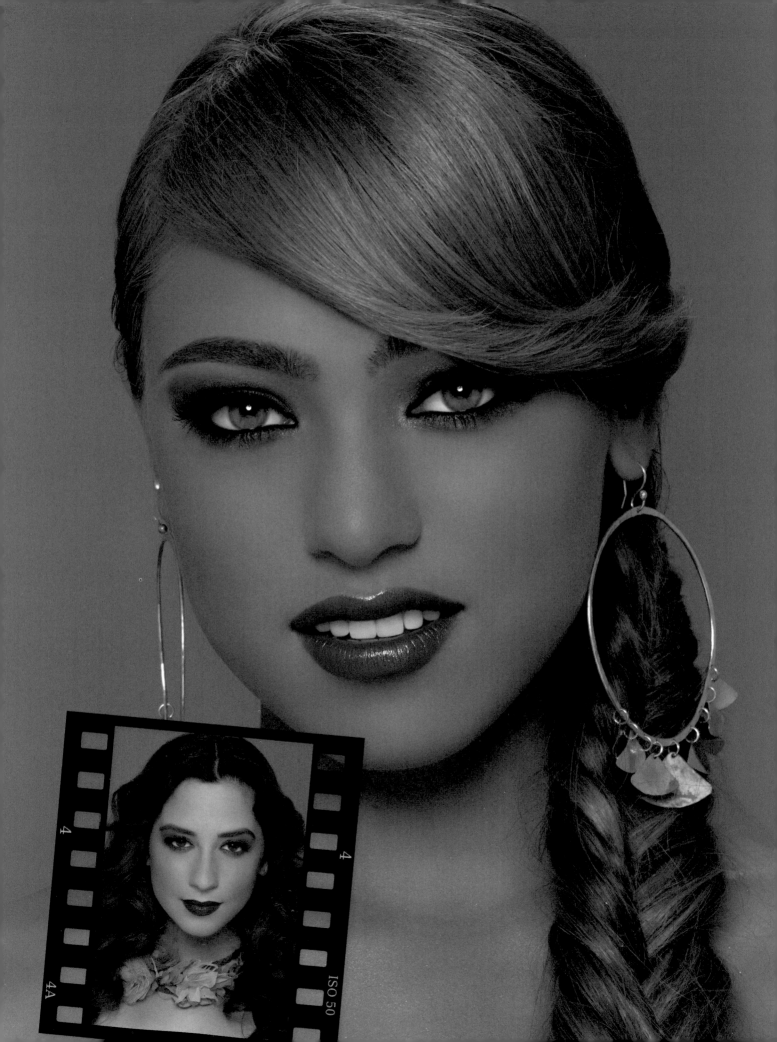

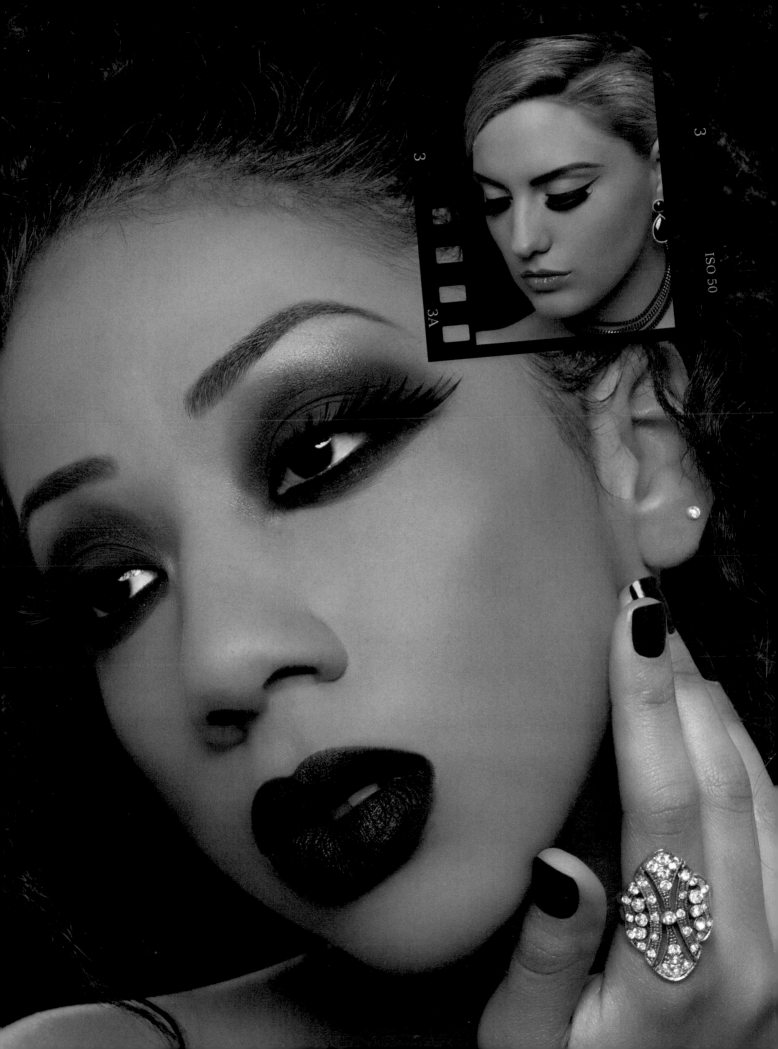

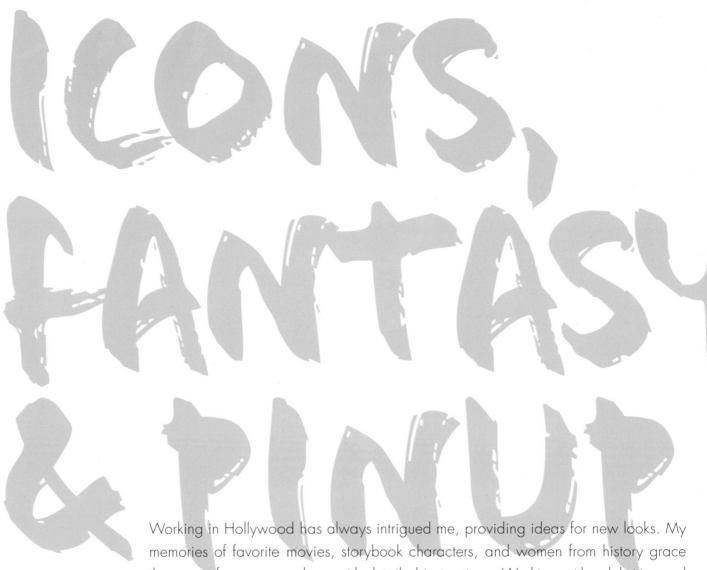

ICONS, FANTASY & PINUP

Working in Hollywood has always intrigued me, providing ideas for new looks. My memories of favorite movies, storybook characters, and women from history grace these next few pages, along with detailed instructions. Working with celebrities and doing their makeup often inspires the characters I create during a show or photo shoot. The personality, profession, and facial features of the individual provide the canvas on which I create. So create your own vignette; start playing and try duplicating one of the looks or change it up to fit your personal vibe for any occasion, from a casual party to something more formal. This section is full of imaginative vignettes demonstrating how makeup helps tell a story.

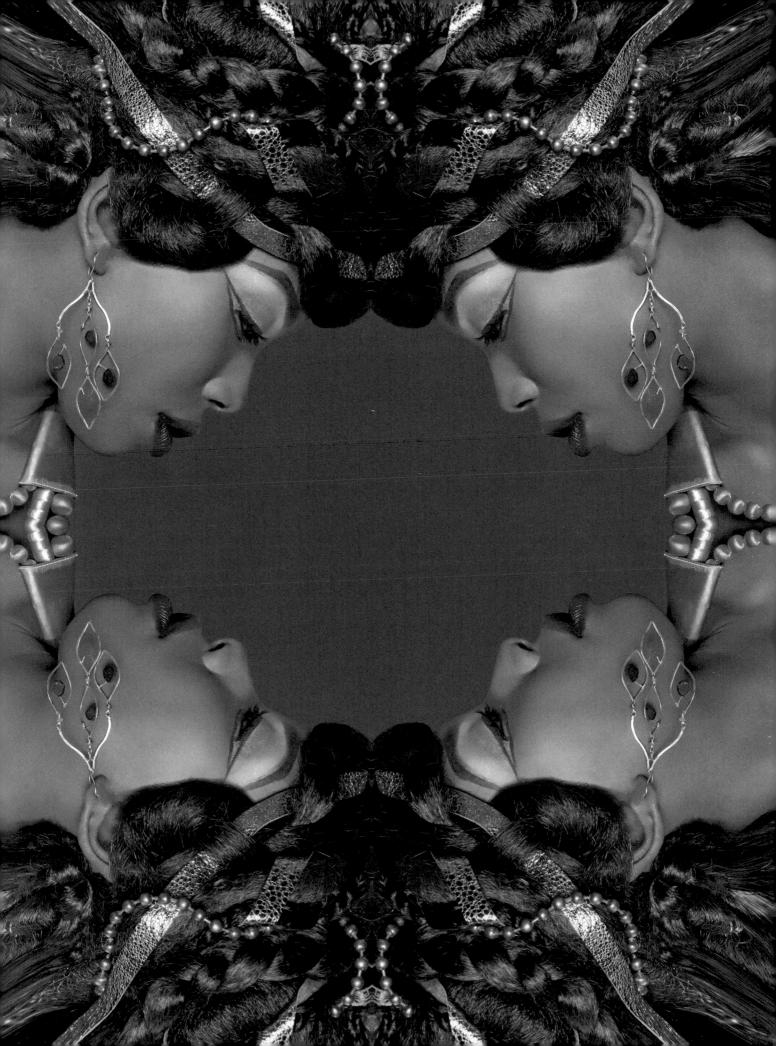

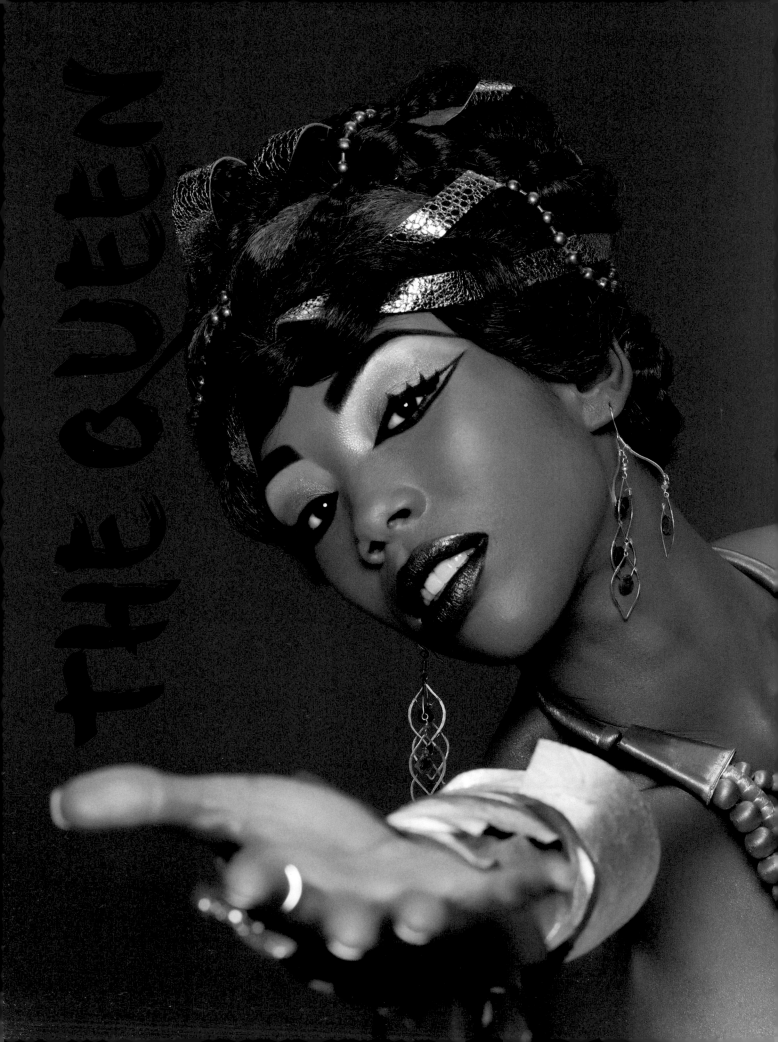

Brandy and I met on *Dancing with the Stars*. She's a graceful and elegant woman. The first image I thought of was Brandy as Queen Nefertiti with her gorgeous long neck and stand-out features. Most people like to try Cleopatra makeup, but Nefertiti doesn't get the same love. I took the challenge and wanted to create something ancient and strong, yet colorful and bright.

* Apply foundation from the eyes up to the forehead and over the eyebrows, blending into the hairline.

* With a wider-than-usual angled eyebrow brush, paint in the brows extra dramatic and thick, using a mix of brown and black gel liner. Paint on brows above the real eyebrows. Draw up and over in an extreme arch, then flare out toward the temple.

* Go over the painted brow with a dark brown eyebrow shadow and angle the brush to soften a bit.

* Apply a bright baby blue cream eye shadow to the lid and up onto the crease using a regular eye shadow brush. Apply a bright lime green cream eye shadow above the crease, rounded all the way out to the end of the brow. With a bright matte yellow cream eye shadow, go from on top of the green to under the brow; blend back in a rounded shape toward the nose and down toward the tear duct.

* Line under the eyes with a black gel liner. As you go toward the outer eye, start creating a space between the liner and the lash line, continuing the line out off the eye as far as the end of the brows. Now line the upper lash line from the tear duct toward the temple, connecting with the bottom liner, creating a triangle that has open space in it. Line around the tear duct as well, pointing extremely toward the nose.

* With a matte yellow loose pigment, go over the yellow cream eye shadow. With a baby blue loose pigment, go over the baby blue cream eye shadow. With a

lime green loose pigment, go over the lime green cream. Blend the pigments with a fluffy eye shadow brush, one for each shade. Use a clean eye shadow brush to blend the edges into each other.

* Apply blue eye shadow under the eye, inside the triangle space of the liner.

* Go back over the black liner.

* Line the inside of the upper and lower waterlines with black gel liner.

* Clean up under the eyes with makeup remover.

* Apply mascara with a small fan brush, followed by another layer of mascara using a mascara wand.

* Apply really big vampy strip lashes with dark Duo.

* Apply foundation to the face, neck, and ears.

* Contour with a dark brown cream color at the jawline using a small foundation brush.

* Apply bronze gold makeup onto the upper cheekbones.

* Blend this all in with foundation brushes and a Beautyblender.

* Powder with a translucent powder.

* Line and fill in the lips with a muted red lip liner.

* Mix black lipstick with a bright yellow lipstick and apply to the lips.

* Mix a light yellow gold and a deep bronze gold body makeup and apply all over the body.

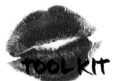

TOOL KIT

FOUNDATION AND CONCEALER

BROWN AND BLACK GEL LINERS

DARK BROWN EYEBROW SHADOW

BRIGHT BABY BLUE CREAM EYE SHADOW AND LOOSE PIGMENT

BRIGHT LIME GREEN CREAM EYE SHADOW AND LOOSE PIGMENT

BRIGHT MATTE YELLOW CREAM EYE SHADOW AND LOOSE PIGMENT

EYE MAKEUP REMOVER

BLACK MASCARA

1 SET BIG VAMPY STRIP LASHES WITH TRIANGLE-SHAPED CLUSTERS

DARK DUO

DARK BROWN CREAM CONTOUR COLOR

BRONZE GOLD BODY MAKEUP

MUTED RED LIP LINER

BLACK LIPSTICK

YELLOW LIPSTICK

LIGHT YELLOW GOLD AND DEEP BRONZE GOLD BODY MAKEUP

FOUNDATION BRUSHES

BEAUTYBLENDER

WIDER-THAN-USUAL ANGLED EYEBROW BRUSH

EYE SHADOW BRUSHES

FIRM POINTY EYELINER BRUSH

SMALL FAN BRUSH

MASCARA WAND

ORANGEWOOD STICK

POWDER BRUSH

LIP BRUSH

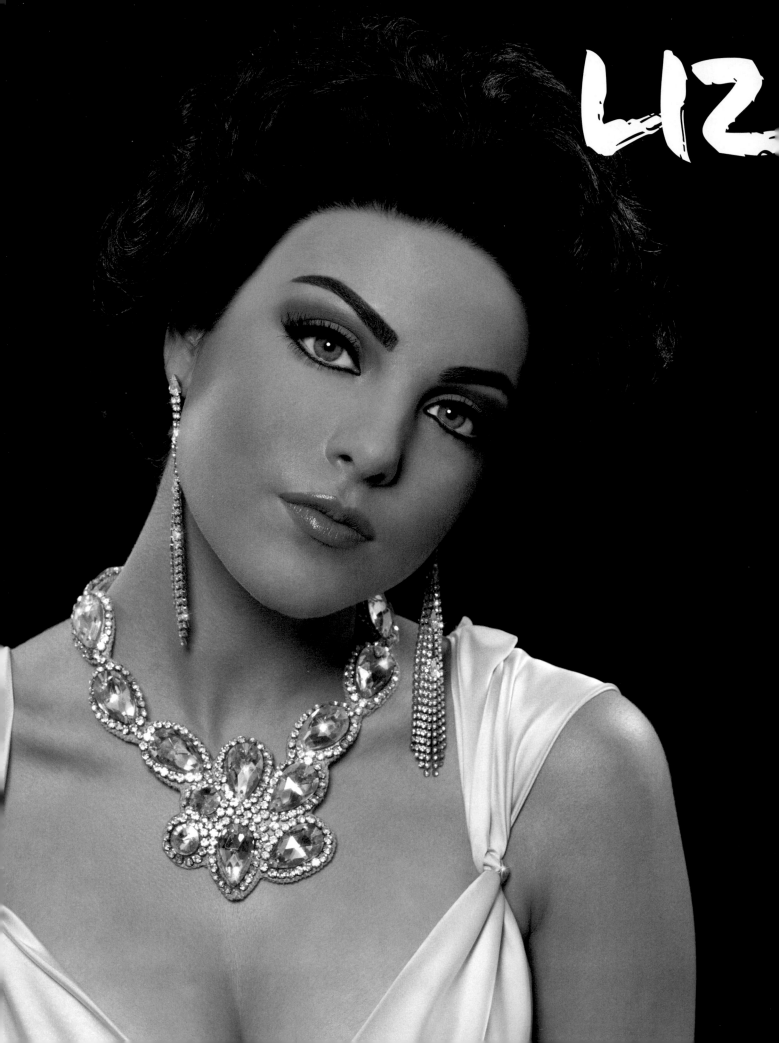

LIZ

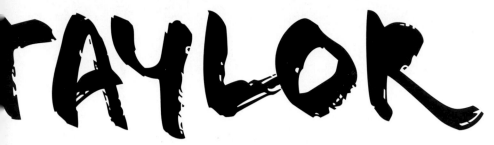

TAYLOR

While we were working together on Nickelodeon's *Victorious*, Liz Gillies and I went through an Elizabeth Taylor phase. She wanted to evoke her spirit, and that is how this shoot was born. We wigged her with the classic Taylor hairdo and had to completely change Liz's skin tone to match Liz Taylor's. When Ms. Gillies walked down the stairs for the shoot, we all felt as if it were Elizabeth Taylor herself.

* Apply foundation to the face, eyes, neck, and ears.

* Contour the nose, jawline, and cleavage with a gray/taupe cream contour color.

* Blend this all in with foundation brushes and a Beautyblender.

* Powder the face with a flesh-colored loose powder; press the powder into the skin using a powder puff to create matte skin. Brush off any excess powder with a brush.

* Perfecting the brows is the key to this look. Liz Taylor was known for her brows. With a wider-than-usual angled eyebrow brush, fill in the brows heavily and define the arch with a dark brown eyebrow shadow.

* Keep the lid clean.

* Apply a matte bone-colored eye shadow from the lid to under the brow, blending in well.

* Apply a matte medium red brown eye shadow to the crease and above, leaving a clean gap between the shadow and the brow.

* With black gel liner, line entirely around the whole eye. The line must be precise. The upper lash line is a definite cat line with a thick tail, connecting under the eye. Line around the tear duct.

* Line the inner upper and lower waterlines with a bone-colored eye pencil.

* Curl the lashes and apply mascara.

* Apply two sets of Demi Wispies lashes with dark Duo.

* Apply mascara again.

* With a blush brush, apply matte pink blush.

* Line the lips with a bright coral pink lip liner. Top off the lips with a thick and luscious bright coral pink lipstick.

* For the body I mixed foundation with a light yellow gold body makeup.

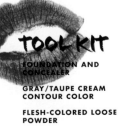

TOOL KIT

FOUNDATION AND CONCEALER

GRAY/TAUPE CREAM CONTOUR COLOR

FLESH-COLORED LOOSE POWDER

DARK BROWN EYEBROW SHADOW

MATTE BONE-COLORED EYE SHADOW

MATTE MEDIUM RED BROWN EYE SHADOW

BLACK GEL LINER

BONE-COLORED EYE PENCIL

BLACK MASCARA

2 SETS DEMI WISPIES STRIP LASHES

DARK DUO

MATTE PINK BLUSH

BRIGHT CORAL PINK LIP LINER

BRIGHT CORAL PINK LIPSTICK

LIGHT YELLOW GOLD BODY MAKEUP

FOUNDATION BRUSHES

BEAUTYBLENDER

POWDER PUFF

POWDER BRUSH

WIDER-THAN-USUAL ANGLED EYEBROW BRUSH

EYE SHADOW BRUSHES

EYELINER BRUSHES

EYELASH CURLER

ORANGEWOOD STICK

BLUSH BRUSH

LIP BRUSH

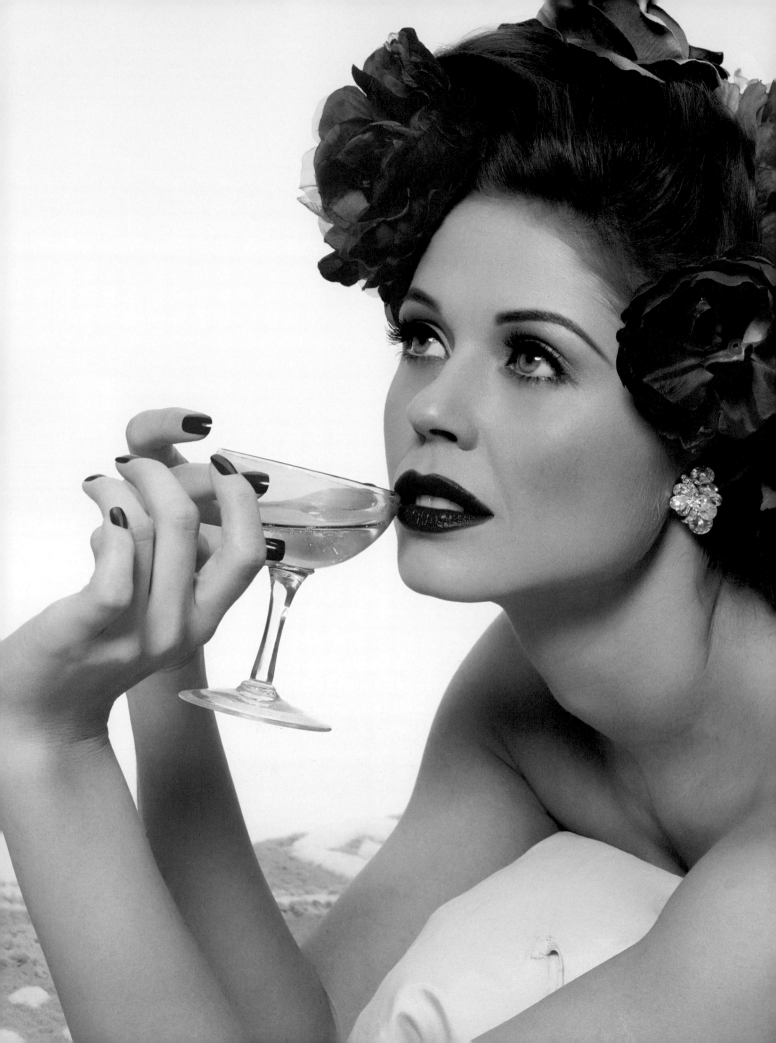

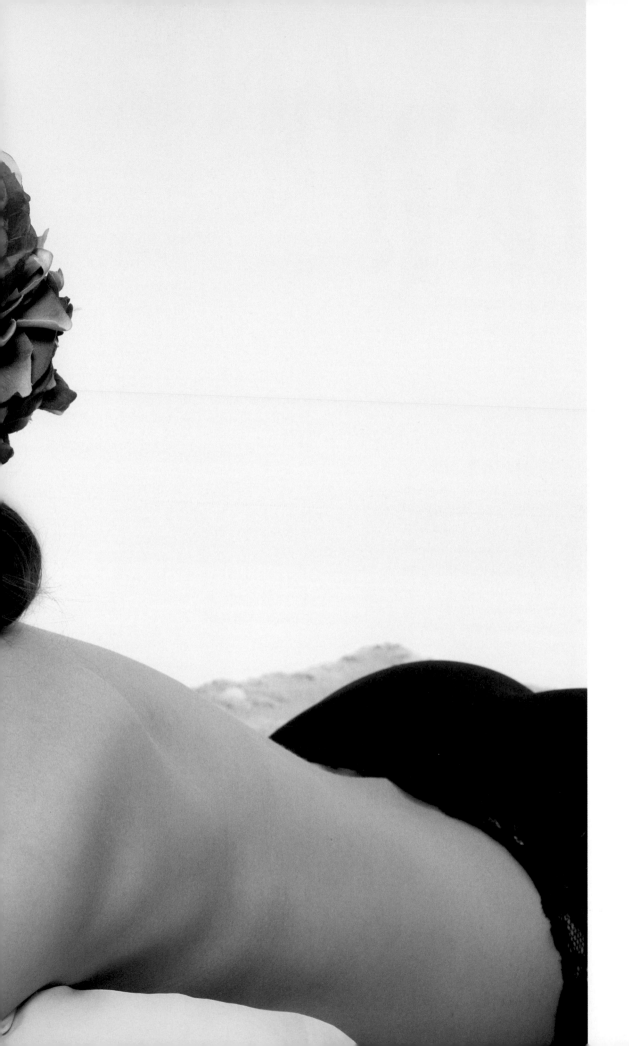

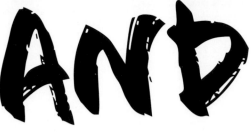

UP, UP, AND AWAY!

It made sense to transform journalist Erin Andrews into a modern Amelia Earhart. An independent woman making history in a field dominated by the other sex: Who better than Erin to represent her? I wanted her makeup fresh and pretty to balance out the boyishness of the outfit. Amelia stood out in her time and was quite fashionable, and you can be too! This timeless look is a perfect daytime work look or for attending a wedding.

* Apply foundation to the face, eyes, neck, and ears.

* Contour the nose and jawline with a gray/taupe cream color.

* Apply a soft pinky peach cream blush to the cheeks, blending up toward the temple.

* Blend this all in with foundation brushes and a Beautyblender.

* Lightly powder the face with a light peach loose powder. Then press a translucent powder onto the face with a puff. Brush off any excess with a powder brush.

* With an angled eyebrow brush, apply clear wax and a taupe eyebrow shadow to the brows. Fill in naturally, rounding the arch.

* Using an eye shadow brush, apply a shimmering deep peach eye shadow to the lid and the crease, blending up toward the brow at the inner eye.

* With an eye shadow brush, apply a shimmering brown eye shadow to the outer crease and the lid, connecting around under the eye. Blend well.

* Line the upper lash line with black gel liner in a cat line with a tight swoop, using a pointed eyeliner brush.

* Line the inner lower waterline with a bone-colored eye pencil.

* Curl the lashes. Apply mascara using a fan brush.

* Apply two sets of Demi Wispies strip lashes using dark Duo.

* Apply mascara again.

* Using a blush brush, apply sparkly peach blush to the upper cheekbones.

* Line the lips and fill in with a peachy nude lip pencil.

* Top off the lips with a sheer pink lipstick.

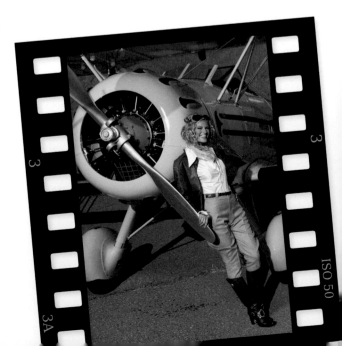

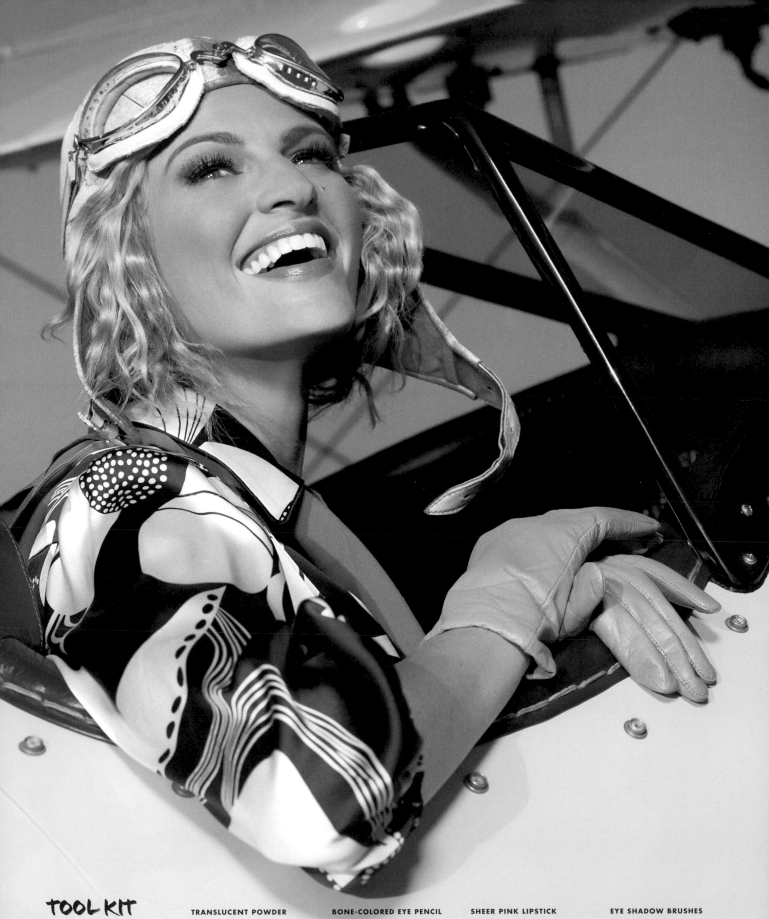

TOOL KIT

FOUNDATION AND
CONCEALER

GRAY/TAUPE CREAM
CONTOUR COLOR

SOFT PINKY PEACH CREAM
BLUSH

LIGHT PEACH LOOSE
POWDER

TRANSLUCENT POWDER

CLEAR WAX AND TAUPE
EYEBROW SHADOW

SHIMMERING DEEP PEACH
EYE SHADOW

SHIMMERING BROWN EYE
SHADOW

BLACK GEL LINER

BONE-COLORED EYE PENCIL

BLACK MASCARA

2 SETS DEMI WISPIES STRIP
LASHES

DARK DUO

SPARKLY PEACH BLUSH

PEACHY NUDE LIP PENCIL

SHEER PINK LIPSTICK

FOUNDATION BRUSHES

BEAUTYBLENDER

BLUSH BRUSH

POWDER PUFF

POWDER BRUSH

ANGLED EYEBROW BRUSH

EYE SHADOW BRUSHES

EYELINER BRUSH

EYELASH CURLER

SMALL FAN BRUSH

ORANGEWOOD STICK

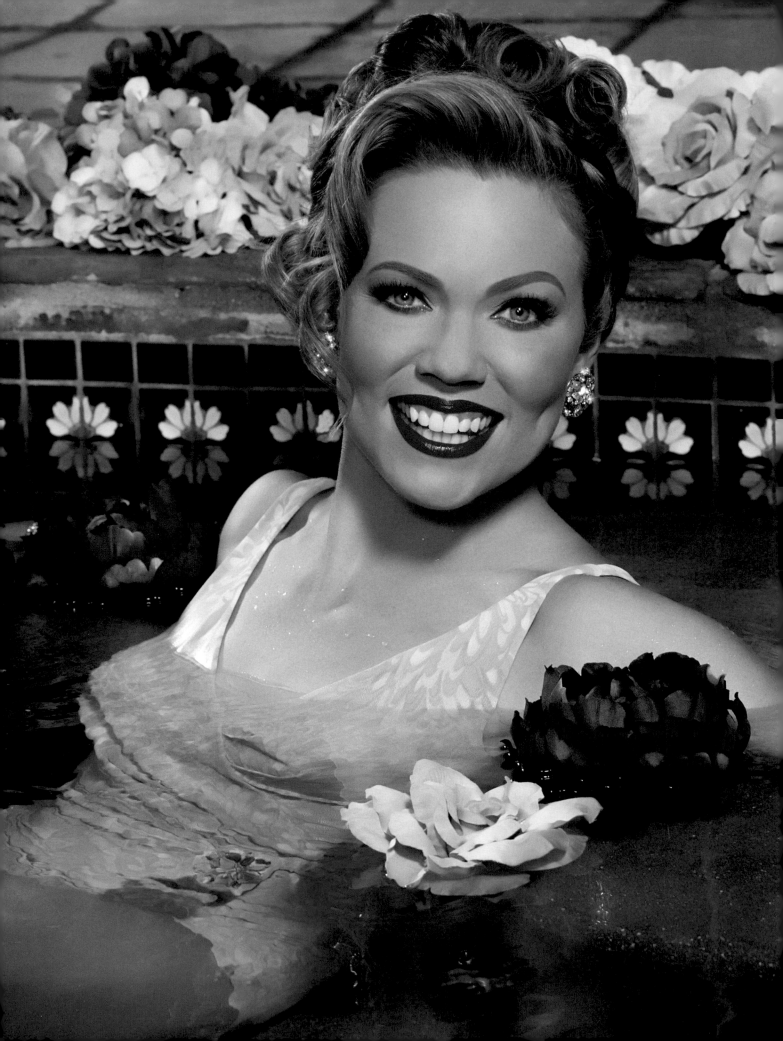

Natalie Coughlin is the first American female athlete in modern Olympic history to win six medals in one Olympics and the first woman ever to win the 100-meter backstroke gold in two consecutive Olympics. Of course I had to do Natalie as Esther Williams, the famous swimmer/movie star of the forties and fifties. This is a classic pinup look; it's timeless and can be worn for any formal event.

* Apply foundation to the face, eyes, neck, and ears.

* Contour under the cheekbones, at the temples, down the sides of the nose, and on the jawline with a gray/taupe cream contour color.

* Apply a sheer red cream blush to the cheeks.

* Blend this all in with foundation brushes and a Beautyblender.

* Dust translucent powder all over the face and press the powder in with a powder puff, fluffing off the excess with a powder brush.

* With a medium brown eyebrow pencil, draw on eyebrows with a full rounded arch, extending the brow end toward the temple.

* Go over the brows with an angled eyebrow brush and medium brown eyebrow shadow.

* Using an eye shadow brush, apply a shimmery cream-colored eye shadow all over the eye from the lid to under the brow.

* With a small eye shadow brush, apply a shimmery light brown eye shadow to the outer crease. With a clean shadow brush, blend the contour toward the inner eye.

* Line under the eye with a shimmery rich brown eye shadow and a blunt fluffy eyeliner brush.

* Using a black gel liner, line the upper lash line with the classic cat line, starting thin at the tear duct and getting thicker toward the swoop.

* Curl the lashes and apply mascara.

* Apply two sets of Demi Wispies strip lashes with dark Duo.

* Apply mascara again.

* Line the inner lower waterline with a bone-colored eye pencil.

* Apply a soft matte baby pink blush on the cheeks with a blush brush.

* Line the lips, slightly overdrawing the top lip, then filling in the lips with a bright cherry red lip liner.

* Apply a creamy candy apple red lipstick.

* Top off the lips with a hot pink lip gloss.

* Mix light yellow gold and rose gold body makeup together and apply all over the body.

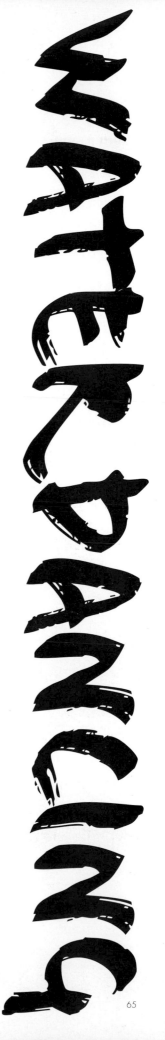

TOOL KIT

FOUNDATION AND CONCEALER

GRAY/TAUPE CREAM CONTOUR COLOR

SHEER RED CREAM BLUSH

TRANSLUCENT POWDER

MEDIUM BROWN EYEBROW PENCIL

MEDIUM BROWN EYEBROW SHADOW

SHIMMERY CREAM-COLORED EYE SHADOW

SHIMMERY LIGHT BROWN EYE SHADOW

SHIMMERY RICH BROWN EYE SHADOW

BLACK GEL LINER

BLACK MASCARA

2 SETS DEMI WISPIES STRIP LASHES

DARK DUO

BONE-COLORED EYE PENCIL

SOFT MATTE BABY PINK MATTE BLUSH

BRIGHT CHERRY RED LIP LINER

CREAMY CANDY APPLE RED LIPSTICK

HOT PINK LIP GLOSS

LIGHT YELLOW GOLD BODY MAKEUP

ROSE GOLD BODY MAKEUP

FOUNDATION BRUSHES

BEAUTYBLENDER

POWDER PUFF

POWDER BRUSH

ANGLED EYEBROW BRUSH

EYE SHADOW BRUSHES

EYELINER BRUSHES

SMALL FAN BRUSH

EYELASH CURLER

ORANGEWOOD STICK

BLUSH BRUSH

LIP BRUSH

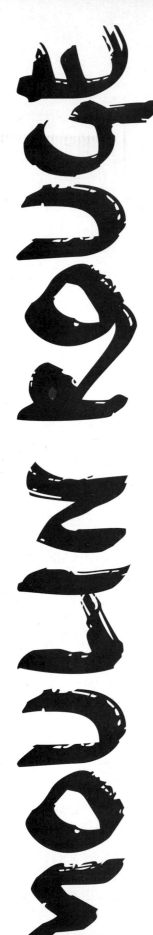

ROUGE MOULIN

Brandy is an amazing singer, actor, dancer, and person. *Elle a une belle ame.* When I found out that Brandy was going to shoot with me, I knew she could embody the famous Josephine Baker. I styled this image from a René Gruau lithograph called "Lido Bonjour la nuit" that I have hanging on my wall, which to me embodies the style and feel of Josephine Baker. I was just waiting for the right girl to stumble into my modern version of the print. I was lucky enough to find an original Lido showgirl costume, on which we sewed fifty beautiful ostrich boas. . . . It was magical! This is another timeless look that is perfect for going to see a show or making a statement while ringing in the New Year.

* Apply foundation to the face, eyes, neck, and ears.

* Contour from the eyebrow down the sides of the nose, under the jawline, and in the hollow under the upper cheekbones, using a dark brown contour color.

* Apply a bright red cream blush to the cheeks up toward the temples; to give a good flush, create a big circle at the apples of the cheeks and blend in.

* Blend this all in with foundation brushes and a Beautyblender.

* With a powder puff, powder the face with a deep peach loose powder. Brush off any excess with a powder brush.

* Using an angled eye shadow brush with clear wax and a dark brown eyebrow shadow, draw a beautiful arch; keep the brow lighter toward the beginning, getting darker and more defined from arch to end.

* With an eye shadow brush, apply a white shimmery loose pigment to the lid and the crease from the tear duct to under the brow.

* Using a crease eye shadow brush, apply a rich brown loose pigment to the outer crease, blending up and out. Use a clean eye shadow brush to blend to ensure a beautiful fade.

* Line the upper lash line with a heavy cat line using black gel liner and an eyeliner brush. Line the inside lower waterline as well.

* Curl the lashes and apply mascara.

* Apply two sets of really plush strip lashes, one different from the other, to create texture, using dark Duo.

* Apply mascara again.

* Go over the lash line with black gel liner. This intensifies and helps to hide the band.

* Apply a matte red blush to the apples of the cheeks, blending up with a blush brush.

* Line the lips and fill in with a cranberry red lip liner.

* Apply a creamy ruby red lipstick.

* Apply a deep bronze gold body makeup all over the body and a touch on the upper cheekbones.

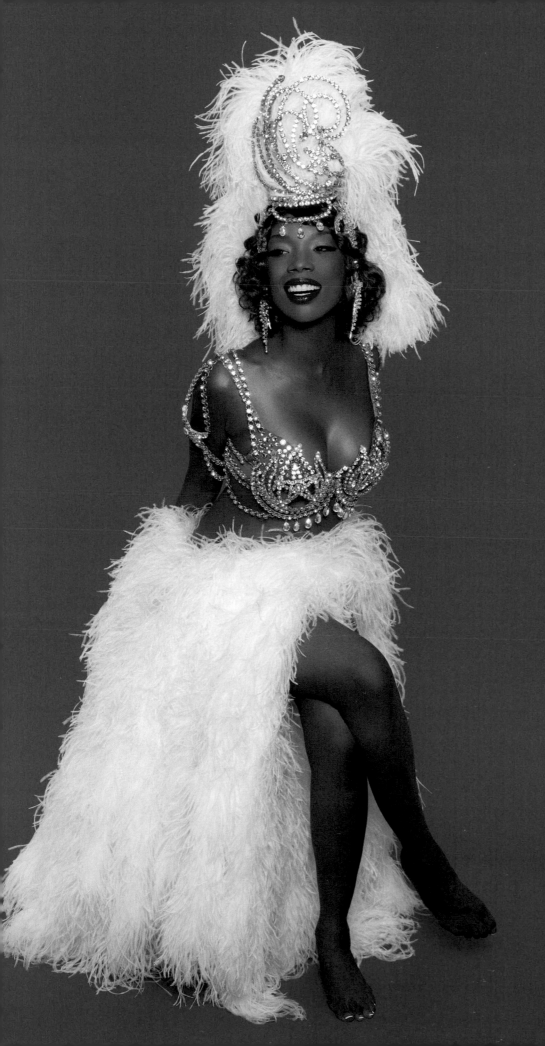

TOOL KIT

FOUNDATION AND
CONCEALER

DARK BROWN CREAM
CONTOUR COLOR

BRIGHT RED CREAM BLUSH

DEEP PEACH LOOSE POWDER

CLEAR WAX AND DARK
BROWN EYEBROW SHADOW

WHITE SHIMMERY LOOSE
PIGMENT

RICH BROWN LOOSE
PIGMENT

BLACK GEL LINER

BLACK MASCARA

2 SETS PLUSH STRIP LASHES,
EACH DIFFERENT

DARK DUO

MATTE RED BLUSH

CRANBERRY RED LIP LINER

CREAMY RUBY RED LIPSTICK

DEEP BRONZE GOLD BODY
MAKEUP

FOUNDATION BRUSHES

BEAUTYBLENDER

BLUSH BRUSH

POWDER PUFF

POWDER BRUSH

ANGLED EYEBROW BRUSH

EYE SHADOW BRUSHES

EYELINER BRUSHES

EYELASH CURLER

SMALL FAN BRUSH

LIP BRUSH

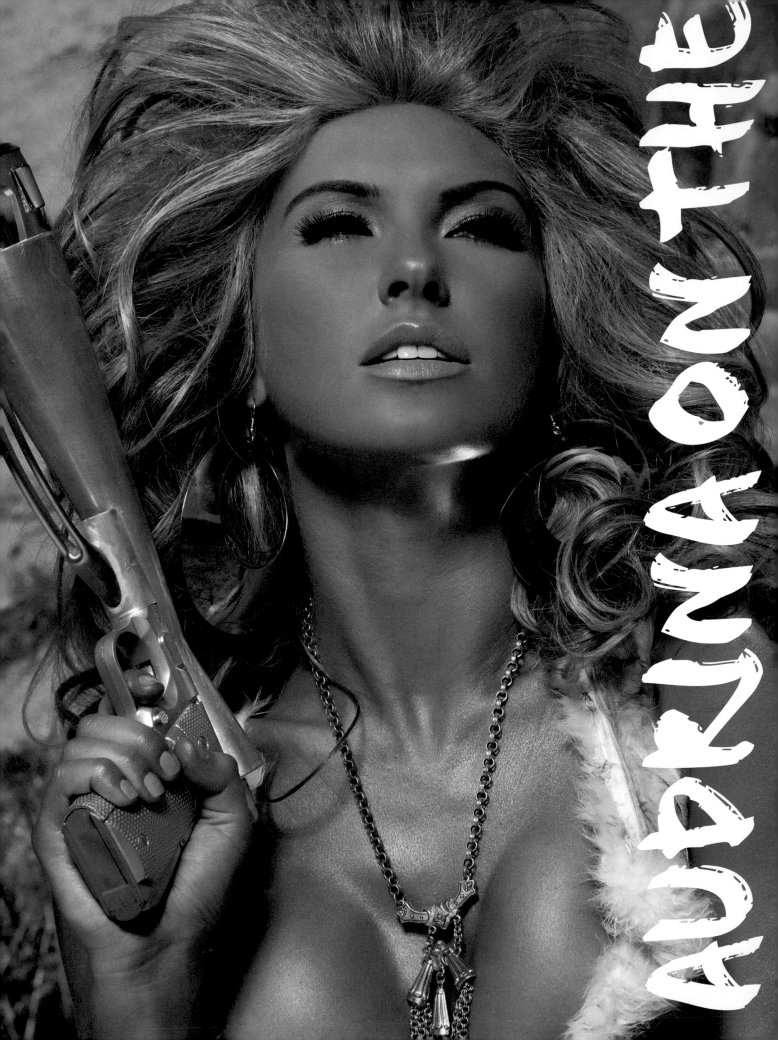

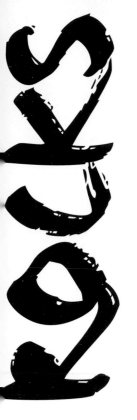

Audrina is an absolute sweetheart. She has gorgeous, flawless skin and quite the body. I always love working with her. Here she is as Raquel Welch from *One Million Years B.C.* Audrina had just gotten back from Australia the day before, and it was one of those fiery hot days in L.A. We took these gorgeous shots of her as a very sexy cavegirl, using the sunburned La Crescenta Hills as background.

TOOL KIT

MATTE LIQUID FOUNDATION
AND BRONZE LIGHT GOLD
AND DEEP GOLD MAKEUP

GRAY/TAUPE CREAM
CONTOUR COLOR

NUDE PINK CREAM BLUSH

YELLOW GOLD MAKEUP

TRANSLUCENT POWDER

CLEAR WAX AND DARK
BROWN EYEBROW SHADOW

MATTE WHITE EYE SHADOW

SHIMMERY CHAMPAGNE
NUDE EYE SHADOW

MATTE BROWN TAUPE EYE
SHADOW

BONE-COLORED EYE PENCIL

BLACK MASCARA

BLACK GEL LINER

2 SETS DEMI WISPIES STRIP
LASHES

DARK DUO

BABY PINK BLUSH

BRONZE GOLD LOOSE
POWDER

VERY PALE PINK LIPSTICK

BRONZE GOLD AND DEEP
GOLD BODY MAKEUP

SHIMMERY BRONZE GOLD
LOOSE POWDER

FOUNDATION BRUSHES,
REGULAR AND SMALL

BEAUTYBLENDER

BODY BRUSH

POWDER BRUSH

ANGLED EYEBROW BRUSH

EYE SHADOW BRUSHES

EYELASH CURLER

SMALL FAN BRUSH

BLUSH BRUSH

LIP BRUSH

* Apply matte liquid foundation that is mixed with bronze light gold and deep glow makeup all over the eyes, face, lips, and ears and down the neck to the chest.

* Contour the jawline, the sides of the forehead, and under the cheekbones with a gray/taupe cream contour color.

* Apply a nude pink cream blush to the upper cheekbones.

* Highlight on top of the brow bones and cheekbones and under the bottom lip in the center of the chin using a yellow gold makeup.

* Blend this all in with foundation brushes and a Beautyblender.

* Powder the face with translucent powder and a powder brush.

* Use clear wax, dark brown eyebrow shadow, and an angled eyebrow brush to make the brows thicker and longer with a rounded arch.

* Apply matte white eye shadow to the lid with an eye shadow brush. Apply shimmery champagne nude eye shadow over the lid to the crease, up to the brow, and then under all of the eye as well.

* Use a slim crease brush to apply matte brown taupe eye shadow to the crease, creating a slight contour.

* Use a bone-colored eye pencil to line the inner lower waterline.

* Curl the lashes and apply mascara.

* Tightly line the top of the lash line with a cat line, and connect down to the lower corner of the eye with black gel liner.

* Apply two sets of Demi Wispies strip lashes using dark Duo.

* With a blush brush, apply a baby pink blush to the cheekbones.

* Sweep bronze gold loose powder across the upper cheekbones.

* Apply a very pale pink lipstick all over the lips.

* Apply bronze gold and deep gold body makeup, mixed, all over the body. For extra oomph, apply a shimmery bronze gold loose powder to the shoulders and cleavage and down the sides of the thighs.

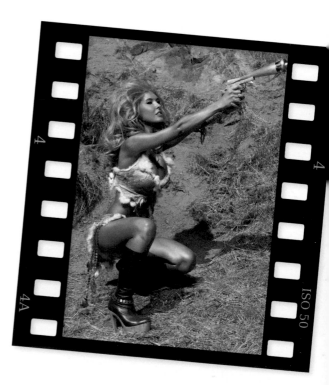

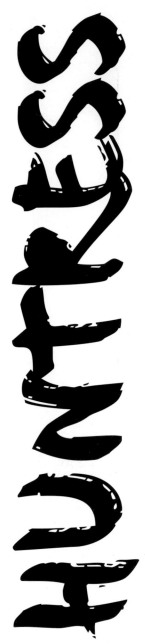

I put an installation together for Concept Fashion Week L.A. in 2011. Working with designer Summer Rose, we came up with the Ice Huntress. Here's the story: Amazon warriors are left to survive on magic after the world has frozen over. I wanted, therefore, a raw, tribal, witchy, yet sexy vibe. The three looks are slightly varied for each girl. It really came alive. For these looks the makeup is relatively simple to achieve and can certainly be repurposed in a less extreme way for a night on the town. Simply leaving out the contacts really tones down the vibe of the makeup.

* Apply Gleam body makeup in shades to match the skin tone all over the body.

* Apply foundation mixed with the body makeup to the face, eyes, neck, and ears.

* Heavily contour the cheeks and under the jaw with a taupe/gray or brown cream contour color.

* Blend this all in with foundation brushes and a Beautyblender.

* Using a fluffy eyeliner brush, line around the eyes with a matte earthy brown eye shadow.

* Contour the eye crease with a matte taupe or brown eye shadow and a small shadow crease brush.

* You can choose to use liner or not. On one of the girls I lined only the inner

upper and lower waterlines with a black gel liner, while on another I lined only the upper lash line.

* Fill in the eyebrows naturally with an angled brow brush, wax, and dark brown shadow.

* Lightly apply black mascara using a small fan brush; don't add fake lashes.

* Apply white shimmery loose powder with blue undertones on the lids, under the eyes, and on the upper cheekbones, the tops of the shoulders, and the collarbone.

* For the lips, use nude or black lipstick. On the center of the lower lip, tap a dash of the same white shimmery powder used on the eyes.

TOOL KIT

GLEAM DEEP BRONZE, LIGHT GOLD, AND ROSE GOLD BODY MAKEUP

FOUNDATION AND CONCEALER

TAUPE/GRAY OR BROWN CREAM CONTOUR COLOR

MATTE EARTHY BROWN EYE SHADOW

MATTE TAUPE OR BROWN EYE SHADOW

BLACK GEL LINER

CLEAR WAX AND DARK BROWN EYEBROW SHADOW

BLACK MASCARA

WHITE SHIMMERY LOOSE POWDER WITH BLUE UNDERTONES

NUDE OR BLACK LIPSTICK

FOUNDATION BRUSHES, REGULAR AND SMALL

BEAUTYBLENDER

LOOSE BIG EYE SHADOW BRUSHES

EYELINER BRUSHES

ANGLED EYEBROW BRUSH

SMALL FAN BRUSH

BLUSH BRUSH

LIP BRUSH

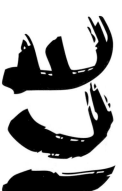

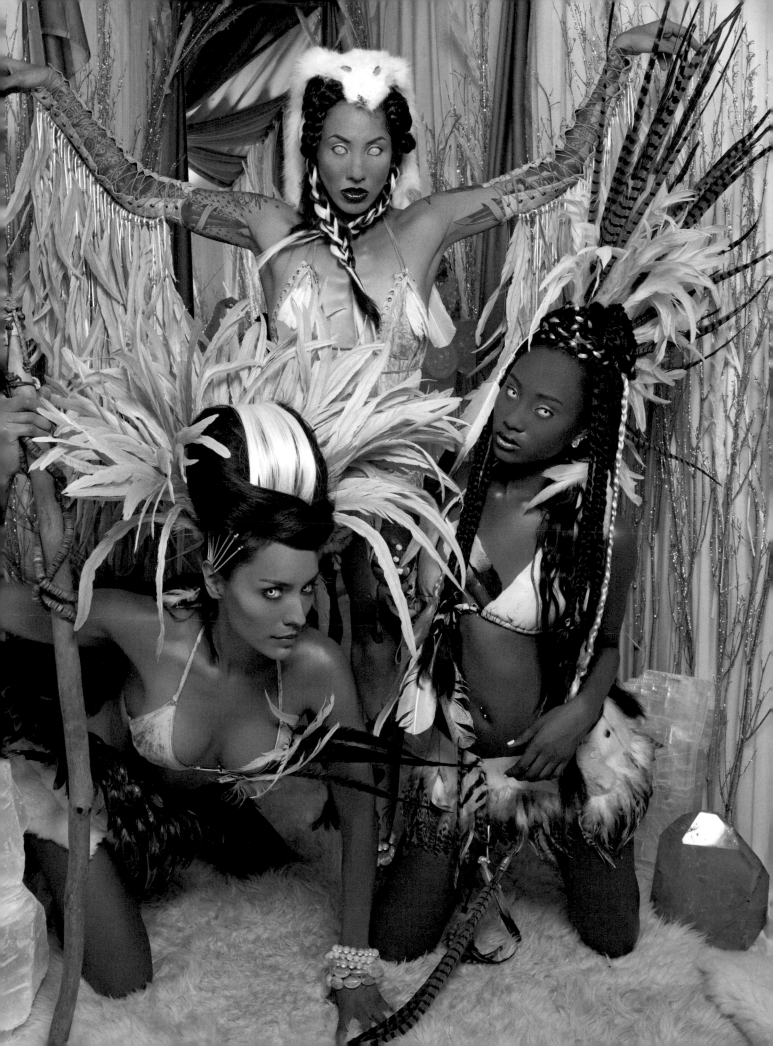

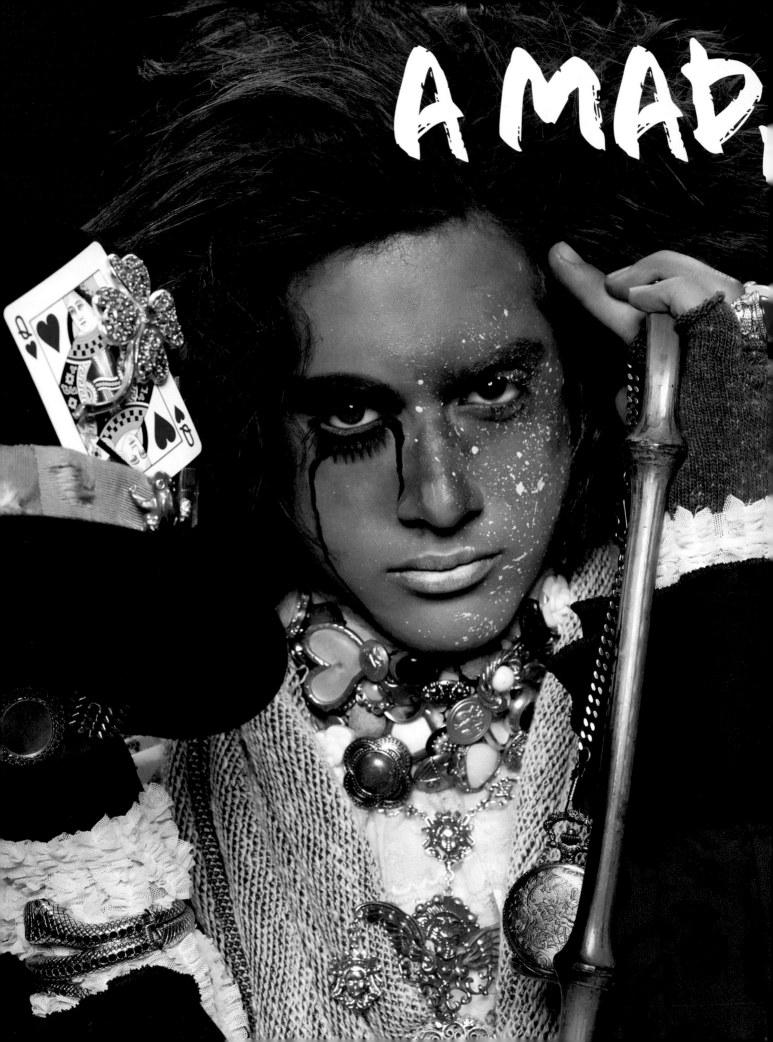

AMAD

MAD HATTER

Avan Jogia is one of America's teenage heartthrobs. He was game for anything and definitely charmed me. Keeping with the theme of what I had done with other *Victorious* actors, I picked a cartoon/storybook icon, choosing the Mad Hatter for Avan. Not only does he kind of remind me of Johnny Depp, but the Mad Hatter fits his fun, playful personality. Don't worry, this makeup works for girls too! This look can certainly be altered to add drama to a club or concert night. Splatter makeup all over your face and body when the makeup has been done; it will add drama and fun. Of course, you can use whatever colors you desire.

* Apply foundation slightly paler than the skin tone all over the face, eyes, neck, and ears.

* Blend this all in with foundation brushes and a Beautyblender.

* Lightly dust the face with translucent powder.

* This look uses aqua colors in black, kelly green, white, and bright orange. These colors, which are activated by water, can last a long time.

* Rip a latex sponge in half, wet the aqua colors with a spritz of water, and soak up the color with the ripped end of the sponge. Start with the orange color and blot around where desired. Next, take the green color and do the same.

* On the left eye, use an eye shadow brush to apply black cream eye shadow all over the lid up to and into the brow. Wing out the brow toward the temple straight from the arch in a flare, then bring the color down toward the tear duct.

* Line the left eye's inner upper and lower waterlines with a black gel liner and an eyeliner brush.

* Do not apply mascara; keep it edgy and raw.

* Paint the same kelly green aqua color under the eye with a thick eyeliner brush.

* Saturate a stiff, big, synthetic brush with very wet white aqua color, then flip the brush hairs back and let go to splatter onto face.

* Tap the white aqua color onto the lips in a nonuniform way.

* Dampen the black aqua color enough that it is dripping rich color off a slim small eye shadow crease brush. Close one eye and hold the head back, then drip drops of black aqua color from the corners of the eyes, lift the head, and let the drops fall to create Mad Hatter tears.

* Apply a spiky full-strip lash, upside down, under the left eye, using clear Duo. Leave a gap between the false lash and the lash line, creating a gap and a menacing *Clockwork Orange* vibe.

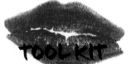

TOOL KIT

FOUNDATION AND CONCEALER

TRANSLUCENT POWDER

BLACK, KELLY GREEN, WHITE, AND BRIGHT ORANGE AQUA COLORS

WATER

BLACK CREAM EYE SHADOW

BLACK GEL LINER

BIG VAMPY STRIP LASH WITH LONG SPIKES THAT ARE SPACED

CLEAR DUO

FOUNDATION BRUSHES

BEAUTYBLENDER

POWDER BRUSH

LATEX SPONGES

EYE SHADOW BRUSHES

SYNTHETIC BRUSHES

EYELINER BRUSHES

ORANGEWOOD STICK

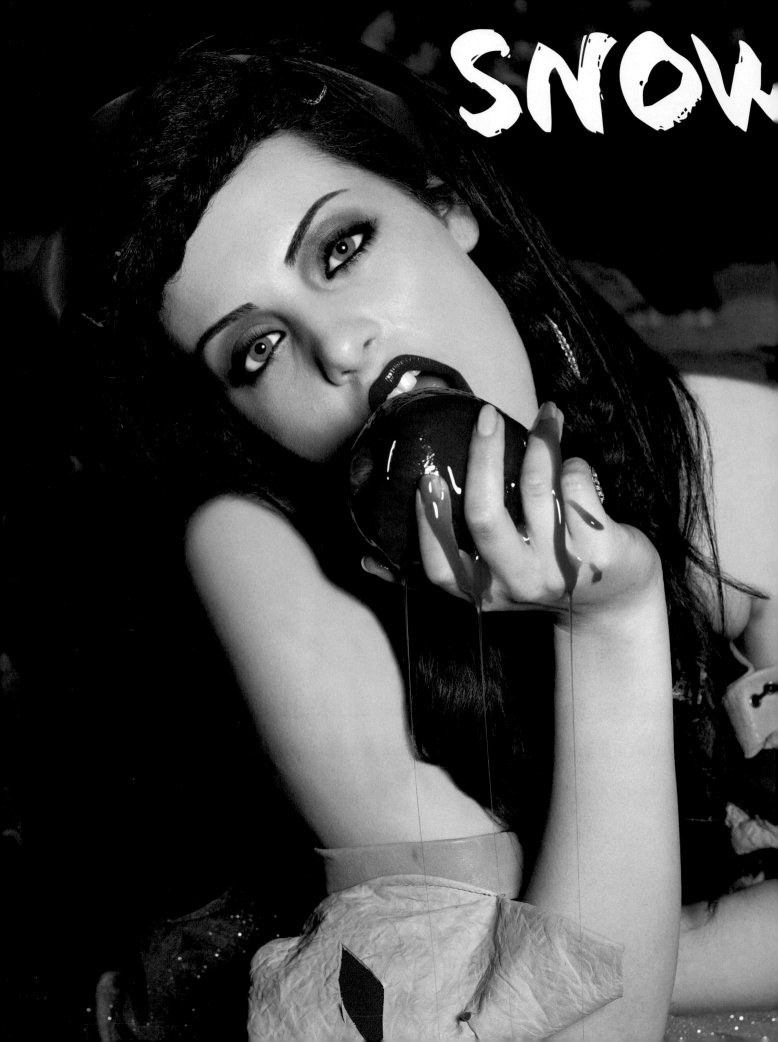

SNOW

WHITE

Liz Gillies reminds me of Snow White with her pale ivory skin, dark black hair (at the time), blue eyes, and stunningly natural red lips. And like Snow White, she bursts out into song all the time. I, of course, wanted something on the edgy side but didn't want her looking like an ad for a Halloween outfit. We designed her costume using handmade varied leather pieces to give edge and added a soft contrast with her flowing long silk and chiffon train. Liz suddenly became a silent movie star playing Snow White. With ragged woodsy hair, her makeup bright and animated, she's that girl with ravishing looks, lost in the woods, running away from the wicked queen. This is stunning makeup that can rock any event.

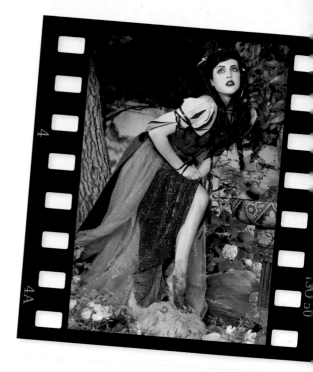

* Apply foundation over the eyes and forehead, blending into the hairline.

* Using a powder brush, lightly powder with a translucent powder.

* Fill in the brows naturally with a medium brown eyebrow pencil.

* Apply cobalt blue eye shadow all over the lid, from the inner tear duct to the outer eye and slightly above the crease in an arch, using a small eye shadow brush.

* Apply an iridescent purple loose pigment to the center of the lid and up toward the crease. Line under the eyes as well, and then blend with a small fluffy eye shadow brush.

* With a small eye shadow brush, apply yellow eye shadow around the tear duct, then blend up into the blue, mixing it all in to create a beautiful peacock effect.

* Take a little of the yellow shadow under the outer brow bone and blend out.

* Line the inner lower waterline with a black gel liner and an eyeliner brush.

* Curl the lashes and apply mascara.

* Layer black individual flare lashes in short, medium, and long along the upper lash line with dark Duo. Layer enough to open the eye while still keeping the lashes natural-looking.

* Apply mascara again.

* Clean up under the eyes with makeup remover.

* Apply foundation to the face, neck, ears, and chest.

* Contour down the sides of the nose and under the cheekbones, using a gray/taupe cream contour color.

* To create a natural flush, apply a sheer red cream blush with a foundation brush to the apples of the cheeks.

* Blend this all in with foundation brushes and a Beautyblender.

* Lightly powder with a translucent powder.

* Line the lips with a cherry red lip pencil.

* Top off the lips with bright red lip gloss, matching the lips to the shade of a poisoned candied apple.

TOOL KIT

FOUNDATION AND CONCEALER

TRANSLUCENT POWDER

MEDIUM BROWN EYEBROW PENCIL

COBALT BLUE EYE SHADOW

IRIDESCENT PURPLE LOOSE PIGMENT

YELLOW EYE SHADOW

BLACK GEL LINER

BLACK MASCARA

BLACK INDIVIDUAL FLARE LASHES IN SHORT, MEDIUM, AND LONG

DARK DUO

GEL EYE MAKEUP REMOVER

GRAY/TAUPE CREAM CONTOUR COLOR

SHEER RED CREAM BLUSH

TRANSLUCENT POWDER

CHERRY RED LIP PENCIL

BRIGHT RED LIP GLOSS

FOUNDATION BRUSHES, REGULAR AND SMALL

BEAUTYBLENDER

POWDER BRUSH

EYE SHADOW BRUSHES

EYELINER BRUSH

SMALL FAN BRUSH

EYELASH CURLER

TWEEZERS

LIP BRUSH

THE WOLF

Daniella Monet, a beauty from Nickelodeon's *Victorious*, is perfect for this dark, saucy Little Red Riding Hood. For my version, Little Red Riding Hood *is* the wolf. She is the witchy seductress who lures innocents into her lair. The makeup is tribal and raw. If you tone down the eyebrows and streaks on the eyes, this look can be worn to rule the night.

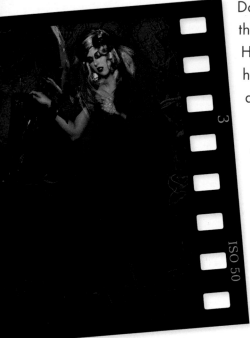

* Apply foundation to the eyes, eyebrows, and forehead and blend into the hairline.

* With a small eye shadow brush, mix a copper cream eye shadow with black gel liner, and, starting from the inner nose near the tear duct, swoop the color up and over the brow, creating a very raw and thick line.

* Apply the copper cream eye shadow all over the lid up to the crease and under eye. Blend a shimmery copper loose pigment on top.

* With an eye shadow brush, apply loose red pigment to the inner corners of the eye, around the tear duct, and under the eye; blend off the eye and toward the hairline.

* With an eye shadow brush, apply a rich sparkly brown eye shadow to the crease; blend around the outer eye connecting to the outer corner under the eye.

* Line the inner lower waterline with a red eye pencil.

* With a black gel liner, line the upper inner waterline and inner tear duct, using an eyeliner brush.

* With a blood-red lip pencil, apply a thin line around the whole eye, then make it extra thick around the outer corner.

* Curl the lashes and apply mascara.

* Apply a set of lush Wispies strip lashes using dark Duo.

* Apply mascara again.

* Clean up under the eyes with makeup remover.

* Apply foundation to the rest of the face, neck, ears, and chest.

* Contour the cheeks, jaw, and neck with gray/taupe cream contour color.

* Apply a red cream blush to the cheekbones all the way toward the outer eye and up toward the hairline.

* Blend this all in with foundation brushes and a Beautyblender.

* Powder just the T-zone with translucent powder.

* With a fluffy blush brush, apply a sparkly red blush to the cheeks, blending up toward the eye.

* With an eyeliner brush, use red lipstick to flare lines off the outer eye, and then across the bridge of the nose and down the sides of the nose.

* Line the lips with a blood-red lip pencil.

* Apply a mix of an eggplant lip gloss and a brick-red lip gloss.

* Apply rose gold body makeup mixed with foundation all over the body.

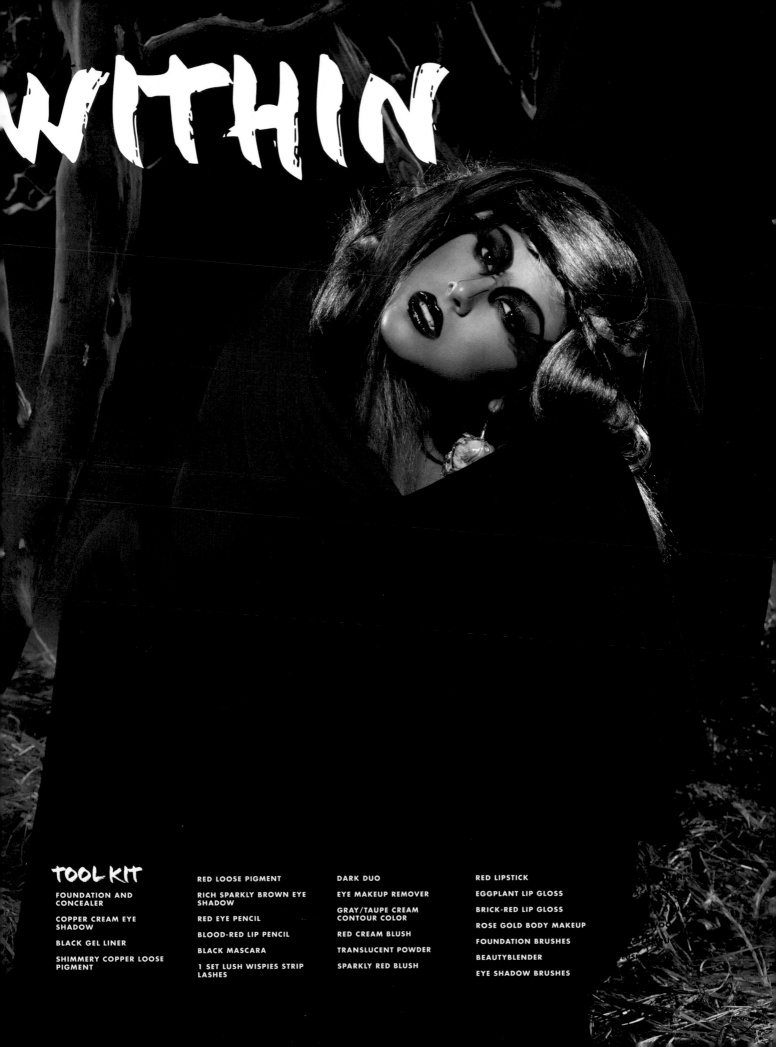

WITHIN

TOOL KIT

FOUNDATION AND CONCEALER

COPPER CREAM EYE SHADOW

BLACK GEL LINER

SHIMMERY COPPER LOOSE PIGMENT

RED LOOSE PIGMENT

RICH SPARKLY BROWN EYE SHADOW

RED EYE PENCIL

BLOOD-RED LIP PENCIL

BLACK MASCARA

1 SET LUSH WISPIES STRIP LASHES

DARK DUO

EYE MAKEUP REMOVER

GRAY/TAUPE CREAM CONTOUR COLOR

RED CREAM BLUSH

TRANSLUCENT POWDER

SPARKLY RED BLUSH

RED LIPSTICK

EGGPLANT LIP GLOSS

BRICK-RED LIP GLOSS

ROSE GOLD BODY MAKEUP

FOUNDATION BRUSHES

BEAUTYBLENDER

EYE SHADOW BRUSHES

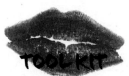

With the help of makeup artist Tyson Fountaine, Aneiska's entire tail was hand-painted and airbrushed. After her hands were done being painted, we glued fabric to her palms to represent webbing. I kept her makeup fresh, natural, and as wet as I could, while still looking glamorous. Of course this look is pure fantasy and extremely dramatic, but be inspired to embellish your body!

For the tail:

* Tyson used first a mix of skin illustrator (alcohol-based liquid colors) of varying colors: blue, silver, black, teal, his own mixes, white, green. He sprayed these through an airbrush, painting in layers all over for the tail, hands, and breasts.

* He then hand-painted layers of like colors using water-based color from MAC and Make Up For Ever. He then locked that all in with more layers of airbrushed alcohol-based colors, finishing off with shimmer powders and glitter.

* Right before the shoot we applied baby oil all over the legs to help give that fishy shine.

For the face:

* Mix a bronze gold makeup into foundation and apply to all of the face, eyes, neck, ears, chest, and upper body. We used no contour; I wanted to keep her face rounded and soft.

* Apply a pink cream blush to the cheeks.

* Blend this all in with foundation brushes and a Beautyblender. Do not powder.

* Brush out the eyebrows. Use an angled eyebrow brush, clear wax, and brown eyebrow shadow to fill in the brows, creating a dramatic rounded arch.

* With an eye shadow brush, apply an iridescent pale blue cream eye shadow all over the lid.

* Using an eye shadow brush, apply a light iridescent blue loose pigment to the inner lid and around the tear duct.

* With an eye shadow brush, apply a bronze brown eye shadow to the outer lid and under the corner of the eye, blending up into the crease.

* Use a blunt fluffy eyeliner brush to apply a rich brown eye shadow all under the eye.

* Mix brown gel liner with a touch of black gel liner and line the upper lash line in a thin tight line using a small pointy eyeliner brush; line the inner tear duct as well.

* Soften the upper lash line by applying a dark brown eye shadow over the gel liner.

* Apply a bone-colored eye pencil to the inner lower waterline.

* Curl the lashes and apply waterproof mascara.

* Lay in individual flare lashes in short, medium, and long with clear Duo.

* Apply mascara again.

* Apply a shiny iridescent blue lip gloss.

For the upper body:

* Before applying anything to the waist and breasts, we applied a rose gold body makeup mixed with bronze gold body makeup all over the upper body.

* Right before shooting, as she was positioned on the rocks, we blew iridescent glitter all over her.

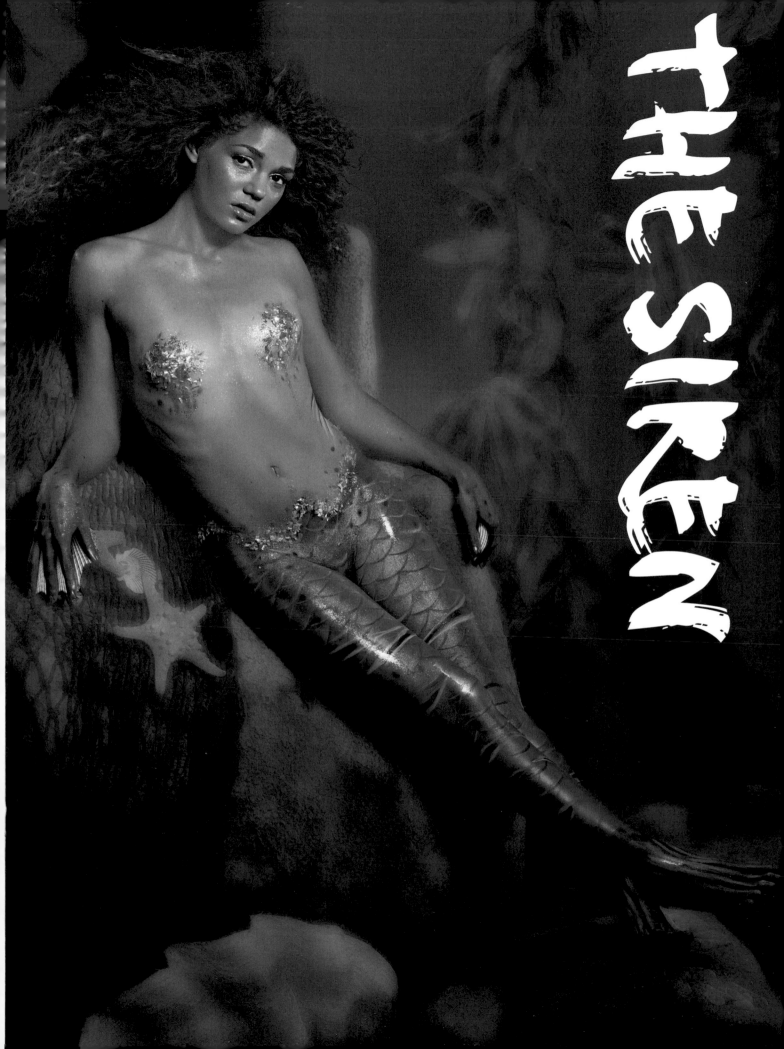

THE SIREN

GLAM

To me glam means big color, be it metallic, smoky, or bright, with big lashes and sometimes a sprinkling of glitter. Above all, being glam means fun! This chapter illustrates how to bring deep drama to your look for a club or party. This is where we play on the wild side—think edgy, sexy, and modern. Smudge your eyeliner for a sultry look; add a bright or metallic gleam to your eye and make your cheeks glow. Think Las Vegas or New York; think the center of attention! The following images should inspire you to be daring. Play with full, lush sets of eyelashes. Try a new, bold color, and don't forget to blast your favorite music to help you get into a creative mood! I hope these looks will spark a fire in your fingers to pick up a makeup brush, grab a pot of colorful loose pigments or some creamy bold eye shadows, and let your inner rock star emerge.

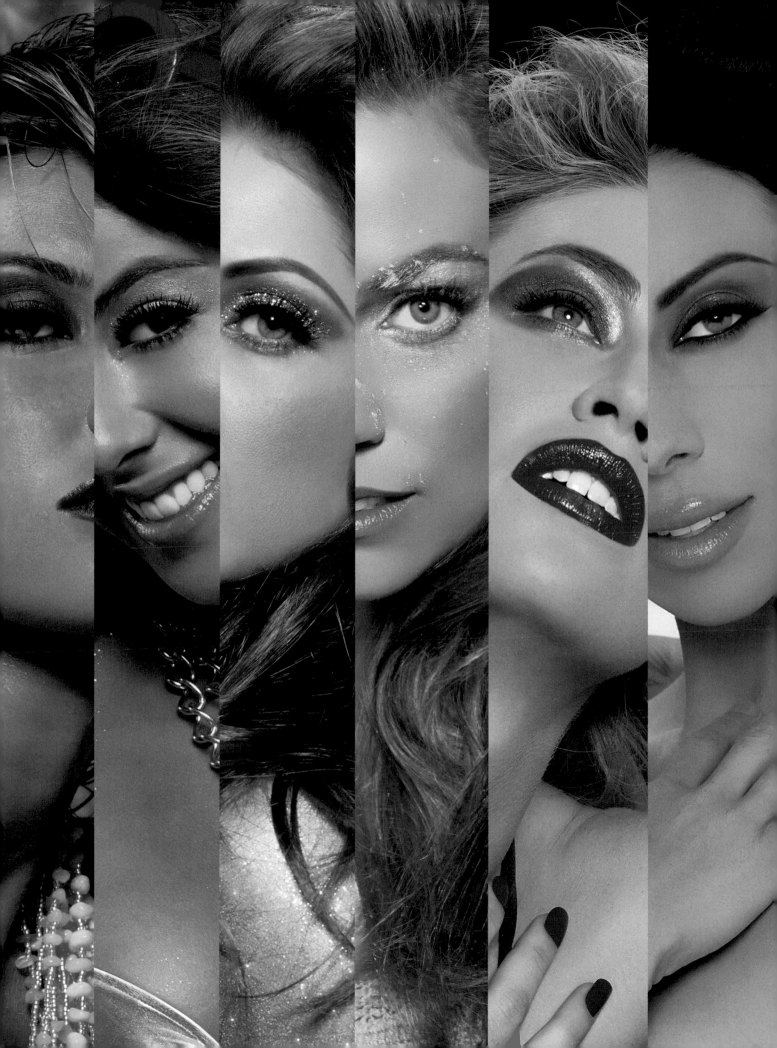

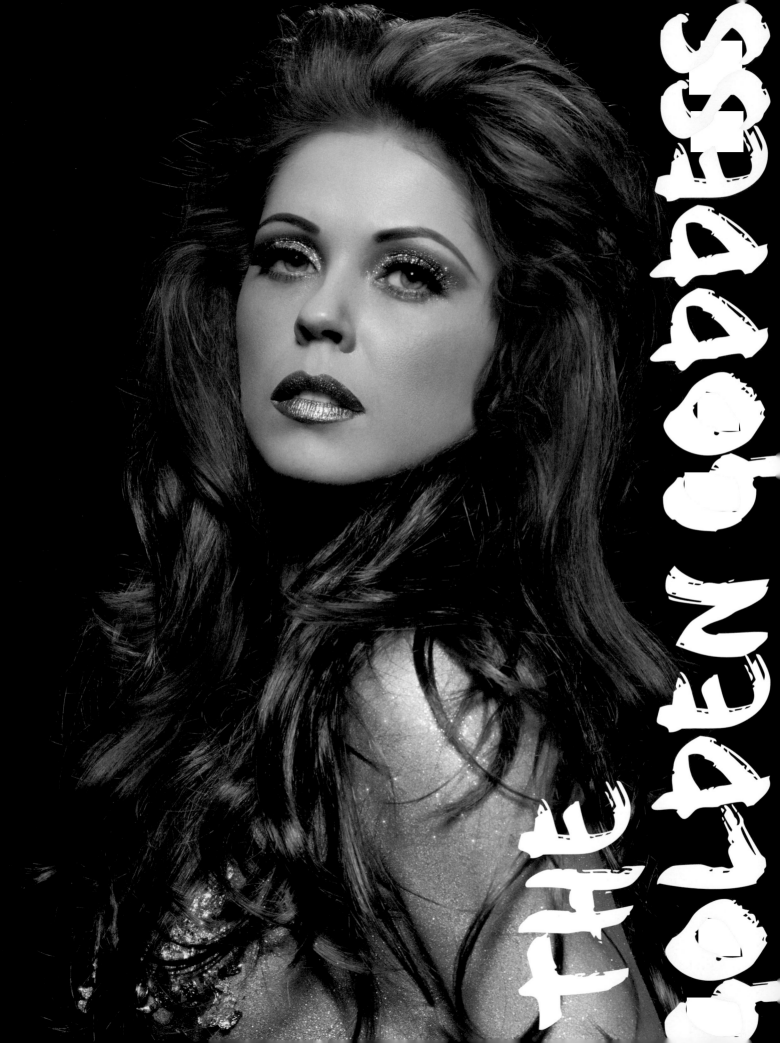

THE GOLDEN GODDESS

I transformed *Dancing with the Stars* ballroom dancer Anna Trebunskaya into a gold and glittering sexy live sculpture. Her sparkling, seductive eyes and red hair perfectly accent her gilded frame. This makeup look is sultry yet fun.

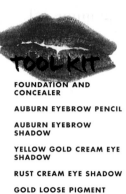

TOOL KIT

FOUNDATION AND CONCEALER

AUBURN EYEBROW PENCIL

AUBURN EYEBROW SHADOW

YELLOW GOLD CREAM EYE SHADOW

RUST CREAM EYE SHADOW

GOLD LOOSE PIGMENT

SPARKLY COPPER RUST EYE SHADOW

BLACK GEL LINER

DARK AND CLEAR DUO

WATER

GOLD GLITTER

GEL EYE MAKEUP REMOVER

BLACK MASCARA

2 SETS PLUSH STRIP LASHES

BONE-COLORED EYELINER

GRAY/TAUPE CREAM CONTOUR COLOR

PEACH CREAM BLUSH

LIGHT YELLOW GOLD MAKEUP

TRANSLUCENT POWDER

ROSE GOLD LOOSE POWDER

YELLOW GOLD CREAM COLOR

YELLOW GOLD LOOSE PIGMENT

GOLD LIQUID BODY MAKEUP

BRONZE GOLD BODY MAKEUP

GOLD LEAF

FOUNDATION BRUSHES

BEAUTYBLENDER

ANGLED EYEBROW BRUSH

EYE SHADOW BRUSHES

EYELINER BRUSH

CERAMIC BOWL

ROUNDED Q-TIPS

TISSUE

SCOTCH TAPE

LATEX SPONGE

EYELASH CURLER

ORANGEWOOD STICK

BLUSH BRUSH

POWDER BRUSH

POWDER PUFF

LARGE FAN BRUSH

For the body:

* Mix gold liquid body makeup, bronze gold body makeup, and gold glitter all together. Apply to clean, dry skin by using a powder puff dipped into the mixture; keep dipping and blending until even. Let dry. Use a Duo wash with clear Duo to adhere gold leaf to the breasts. Tap gold glitter all over the body using a large fan brush.

For the face:

* Apply foundation to the eyes and forehead, blending up into the hairline.

* With an auburn eyebrow pencil, fill in the brow and draw an arch.

* With an auburn eyebrow shadow and an angled eyebrow brush, go over the brow, flaring out the brow ends dramatically.

* With an eye shadow brush, apply yellow gold cream eye shadow to the lids and under the eye, blending around the tear duct.

* Apply rust cream eye shadow to the crease and slightly above; blend out as far as the end of the brow.

* Go over the lid with a gold loose pigment to lock in the color.

* Go over the crease with a sparkly copper rust eye shadow and extend out to the end of the brow; connect under the outer corner of the eye and blend.

* Line the upper lash line with black gel liner.

* Create a Duo wash with clear Duo and water in a ceramic bowl and dip into the mixture with a rounded Q-tip.

* Fold a tissue over the lashes.

* Plunge the Q-tip that has glue on it into gold glitter and tap all over the eyes.

(It's important to keep the eyes closed lightly until the glitter is dry.)

* Remove the tissue and brush excess glitter out of the eyelashes.

* Clean up under the eyes with a triangle latex sponge and gel makeup remover, and use Scotch tape to pick up stubborn glitter.

* Line the upper lash line with another coat of black gel liner.

* Curl the lashes and apply mascara.

* Apply two sets of plush strip lashes with dark Duo.

* Apply mascara again.

* Line the inner lower waterline with bone-colored eyeliner.

* Apply foundation to the rest of the face.

* Contour with gray/taupe cream contour color down the sides of the nose, along the jawline, and under the cheeks.

* Apply peach cream blush to the cheekbones.

* On top of the cheekbones and under the lips, use a light yellow gold makeup to highlight.

* Blend this all in with foundation brushes and a Beautyblender.

* Lightly powder with translucent powder and a powder brush.

* Apply rose gold loose powder on top of the cheeks up to the hairline, and a little on both temples, with a blush brush.

* Apply a mix of yellow gold cream color, yellow gold loose pigment, and gold glitter for the lips.

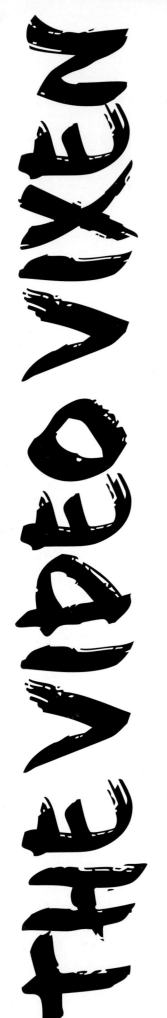

THE VIDEO VIXEN

Jennette McCurdy is a blast. I've had the opportunity to work alongside her on Nickelodeon's *iCarly*. She is really fun and sweet. Her fans enjoy seeing her as the fresh, young sweet thing that she is, but here she's completely opposite: no longer innocent, but a real vixen!

* Apply foundation all over the eyes and forehead and into the hairline.

* Draw in eyebrows with clear wax and a dark brown eyebrow shadow; paint them extra fierce, extending them well past the natural brow.

* With an eye shadow brush, apply bright royal blue cream eye shadow over the lid.

* Lock in the cream eye shadow with a bright deep blue loose pigment applied on top using an eye shadow brush.

* Apply an eggplant/raspberry purple loose pigment from the tear duct to the brow around the inner eye; head toward the nose in a circular motion and then blend out onto the crease to the end of the brow. At the outer eye, use a circular motion to connect to under the eye; line under the eye with shadow. Blend well.

* Clean up under the eyes with makeup remover.

* Line the inner tear duct and upper and lower waterlines with black gel liner; also go along the upper lash line with a very tight line.

* Curl the lashes and apply mascara.

* Apply a set of big triangular-shaped strip lashes using dark Duo.

* Apply foundation to the rest of the face, lips, neck, and ears.

* Contour down the sides of the nose, at both temples, and from under the cheekbones to the jawline to slim the cheeks with a gray/taupe cream contour color.

* Apply a red cream blush on the cheekbones and slightly under.

* Blend this all in with foundation brushes and a Beautyblender.

* Powder lightly with translucent powder, using a powder brush.

* Apply a light plum blush high on the cheekbones with a contoured blush brush.

* Shape the lips by using a cherry lip liner, connecting the upper lip points to give a round shape.

* Once completely shaped, fill in the lips.

* Apply a blue-red lipstick.

* Top off the lips with a hot pink lip gloss.

TOOL KIT

FOUNDATION AND CONCEALER

CLEAR WAX AND DARK BROWN EYEBROW SHADOW

BRIGHT ROYAL BLUE CREAM EYE SHADOW

BRIGHT DEEP BLUE LOOSE PIGMENT

EGGPLANT/RASPBERRY PURPLE LOOSE PIGMENT

MAKEUP REMOVER

BLACK GEL LINER

BLACK MASCARA

1 SET BIG TRIANGULAR-SHAPED STRIP LASHES

DARK DUO

GRAY/TAUPE CREAM CONTOUR COLOR

RED CREAM BLUSH

LIGHT PLUM BLUSH

TRANSLUCENT POWDER

CHERRY RED LIP LINER

BLUE-RED LIPSTICK

HOT PINK LIP GLOSS

FOUNDATION BRUSHES, REGULAR AND SMALL

BEAUTYBLENDER

ANGLED EYEBROW BRUSH

EYE SHADOW BRUSHES, REGULAR AND SMALL

EYELINER BRUSH

EYELASH CURLER

SMALL FAN BRUSH

ORANGEWOOD STICK

CONTOURED BLUSH BRUSH

POWDER BRUSH

LIP BRUSH

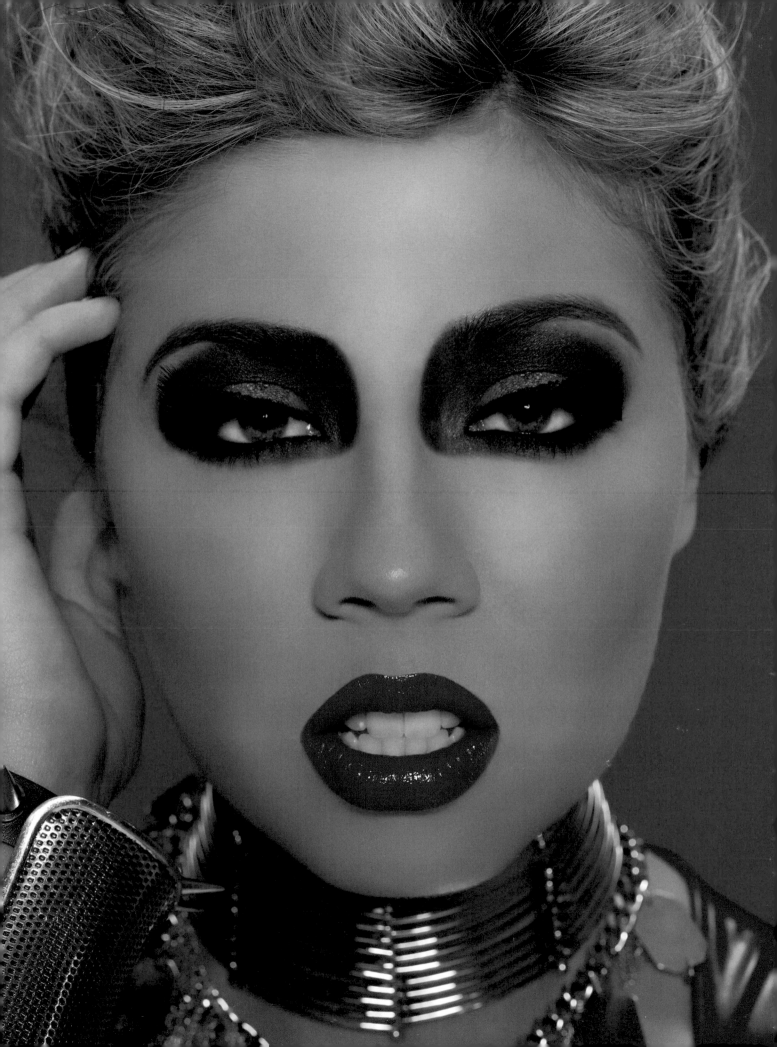

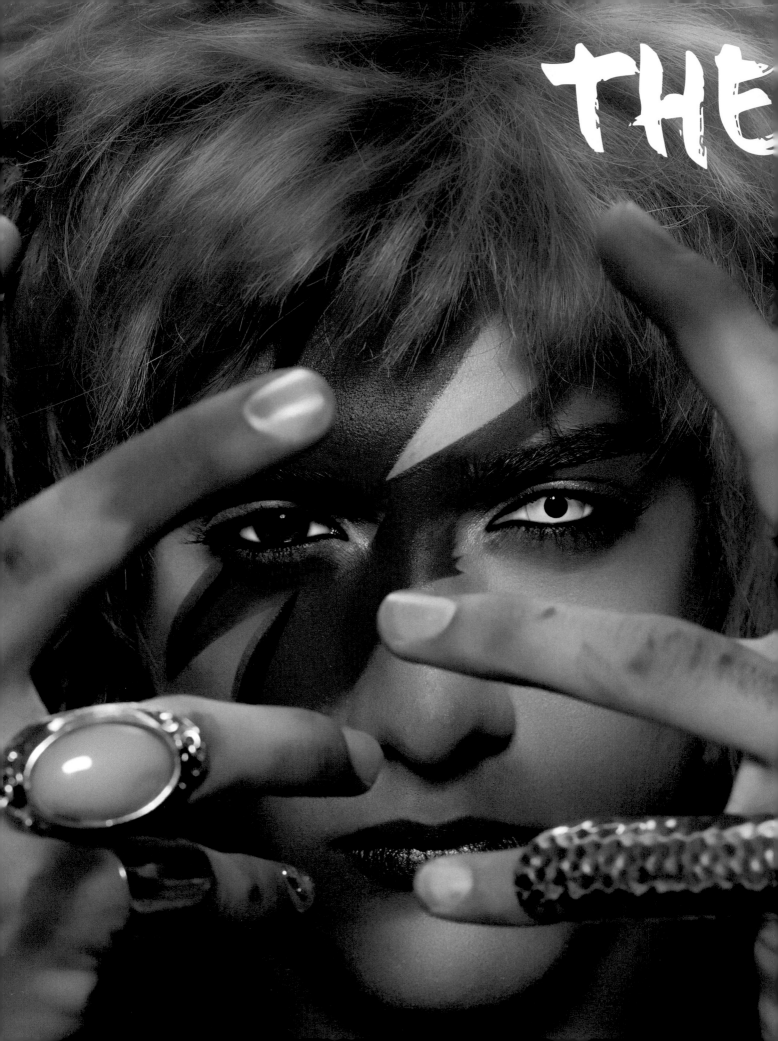

THE

ROCK STAR

One of Avan Jogia's favorite singers is David Bowie; I knew he would make the perfect rock icon. I was inspired by the famous "bolt" Bowie used to sport. This became the perfect makeup centerpiece. I have seen people at the club rocking lightning bolts either on a cheek or like this over the eye. Be creative and use any combo of colors for the bolt on any type of makeup. Decide whether you would like to place a star, moon, or, in this case, a lightning bolt! To put our twist on Bowie's famous eyes, we took it to the extreme by putting a white contact lens in one eye.

* Apply foundation to the skin, eyes, neck, and ears with a foundation that is slightly lighter than the skin tone; this is a pale look.

* Contour from the temples down under the cheekbones using a gray/taupe cream contour color.

* Blend this all in with foundation brushes and a Beautyblender.

* Lightly powder with translucent powder and a powder puff.

* Use a small eye shadow brush to apply gold loose powder to the lid, around the tear duct, and under the eye; blend.

* Line the inner upper and lower waterlines, along with the inner tear duct, using black gel liner and an eyeliner brush.

* Lightly apply mascara with a fan brush.

* Brush the eyebrows.

* Next, paint the first part of the lightning bolt using a red aqua color (color activated by water); using a flat square eye shadow brush, paint the bolt onto the face, avoiding the eye. Outline the red with black gel liner, and then outline the black with a bright blue gel liner. Use various different-size eye shadow and eyeliner brushes for desired thickness of lines.

* Apply copper lipstick to the lips.

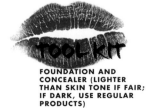

TOOL KIT

FOUNDATION AND CONCEALER (LIGHTER THAN SKIN TONE IF FAIR; IF DARK, USE REGULAR PRODUCTS)	GRAY/TAUPE CREAM CONTOUR COLOR	BLACK MASCARA	FOUNDATION BRUSHES	SMALL FAN BRUSH
	TRANSLUCENT POWDER	RED AQUA COLOR	BEAUTYBLENDER	EYEBROW BRUSH
	GOLD LOOSE POWDER	BRIGHT BLUE GEL LINER	POWDER PUFF	LIP BRUSH
	BLACK GEL LINER	COPPER LIPSTICK	EYE SHADOW BRUSHES	
			EYELINER BRUSHES	

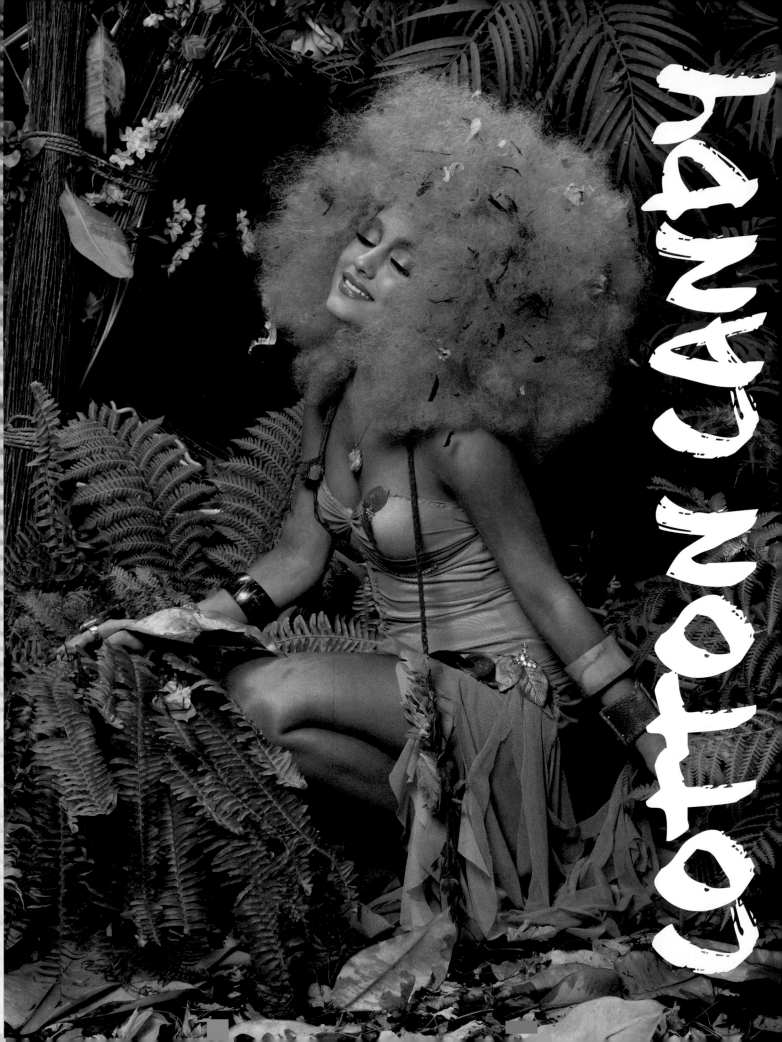

COTTON CANDY

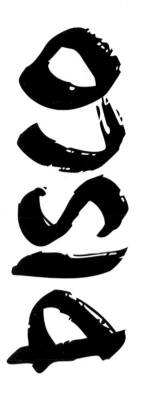

When Ariana and I were discussing which looks to do for her shoot, the one thing she kept saying was, "I want a huge pink Afro!" So here she is as a whimsical wood fairy with a disco sexy edge. Grab a fun wig, put on unique makeup, and hit the town to create a memory other than on Halloween.

* Apply foundation on the lids and up to the forehead into the hairline.

* With an eye shadow brush, apply a mint green shimmery loose pigment all over the lid, toward the nose, and under the eye in a circular motion.

* Apply a yellow gold shimmery loose pigment with an eye shadow brush under the brow to the inner eye, around the tear duct, and under the eye around the green, all the way down to the upper cheekbone in a circular motion. Blend well.

* Use an angled eyebrow brush with clear wax and a taupe eyebrow shadow to lightly fill in the eyes.

* Apply black gel liner inside the upper and lower waterlines, and also tightly on the upper lid, using a small pointy eyeliner brush.

* Curl the lashes and apply mascara.

* Apply a set of Demi Wispies strip lashes with dark Duo.

* Apply mascara again.

* Apply foundation to the rest of the face, neck, and ears.

* Apply a baby pink cream blush to the apples of the cheeks.

* Blend this all in with foundation brushes and a Beautyblender.

* Using a powder brush, lightly dust HD translucent powder over the face.

* Line the lips with a shimmery rose lip pencil. Create a round, fuller upper lip line by overdrawing a bit.

* Top off the lips with a baby pink lip gloss.

* Apply rose gold body makeup all over the body.

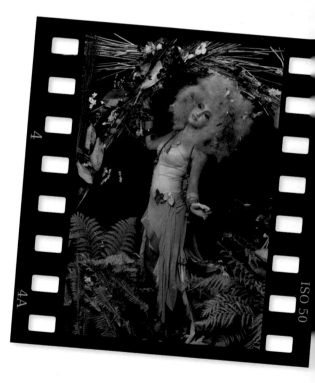

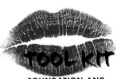

TOOL KIT

FOUNDATION AND CONCEALER

MINT GREEN SHIMMERY LOOSE PIGMENT

YELLOW GOLD SHIMMERY LOOSE PIGMENT

CLEAR WAX AND TAUPE EYEBROW SHADOW

BLACK GEL LINER

BLACK MASCARA

1 SET DEMI WISPIES STRIP LASHES

DARK DUO

BABY PINK CREAM BLUSH

HD TRANSLUCENT POWDER

SHIMMERY ROSE LIP PENCIL

BABY PINK LIP GLOSS

ROSE GOLD BODY MAKEUP

FOUNDATION BRUSHES

BEAUTYBLENDER

EYE SHADOW BRUSHES

ANGLED EYEBROW BRUSH

EYELINER BRUSHES

EYELASH CURLER

SMALL FAN BRUSH

ORANGEWOOD STICK

POWDER BRUSH

LIP BRUSH

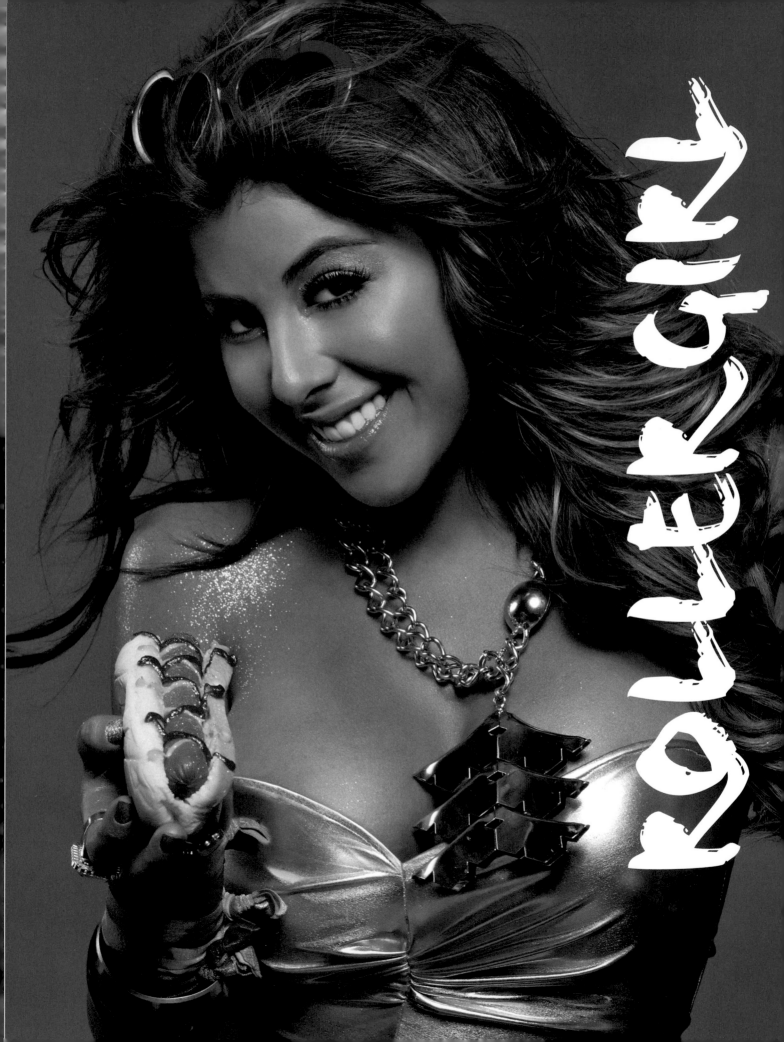

ROLLERGIRL

Daniella Monet has got legs for days! I envisioned her as a roller derby queen from the seventies. Tiny clothes and gold, glittery roller skates made the look.

* Apply foundation to the eyes and forehead and up into the hairline.

* With an angled eyebrow brush, use clear wax and dark brown eyebrow shadow to fill in the brow, amplify the arch, and extend the brow ends.

* With an eye shadow brush, apply a metallic baby blue cream eye shadow all over the lid and up toward the outer crease.

* Apply lavender loose pigment all over the lid and up to the brow with a fluffy eye shadow brush, locking in the cream powder and creating a beautiful color transition.

* Use a small fluffy eye shadow brush and a lime green eye shadow to line around the tear duct.

* With a small eye shadow brush, apply a light shimmery yellow gold loose powder around the tear duct on top of the green, again creating a beautiful color transition.

* Line the upper lash line with a cobalt blue gel liner and tightly line the outer bottom corner, using an eyeliner brush.

* Apply yellow glitter mostly to the inner eye area.

* Create a Duo wash with clear Duo.

* Fold a tissue, then place the folded edge on top of the eyelashes to guard them and catch glitter. Dip a rounded Q-tip into the wash, then tap onto desired areas of the eye; then take the same Q-tip with wash on it and dip it in glitter before tapping onto the eye. Close the eyes lightly and keep them closed to let the glue dry; then use a small fan brush to get all the extra glitter off. Use Scotch tape to pick up unwanted glitter pieces.

* Curl the lashes and apply mascara.

* Apply a set of flirty Wispies strip lashes with clear Duo.

* Apply long individual flare lashes to the outer lash line with clear Duo.

* Line the inner waterlines with a bone-colored eye pencil.

* Clean up under the eyes with makeup remover.

* Apply foundation to the rest of the face, neck, and ears and down onto the chest, mixing a deep bronze gold makeup into the foundation. Also dab a little of the mix above the eyebrow arch.

* Apply a yellow gold makeup to the top of the cheekbones, above the eyebrow, and a touch under the lip.

* Blend this all in with foundation brushes and a Beautyblender.

* Lightly dust the face with translucent powder and a powder brush.

* Apply a shimmery coral blush to the upper cheekbones.

* Apply a baby coral pink lip gloss.

* Spread deep gold body makeup all over the body with your hands; make sure to apply to clean, dry skin.

* Top off with gold rainbow glitter using a big fluffy fan brush; dip the brush in glitter and tap out the glitter onto the desired spots.

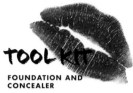

TOOL KIT

FOUNDATION AND CONCEALER

CLEAR WAX AND DARK BROWN EYEBROW SHADOW

METALLIC BABY BLUE CREAM EYE SHADOW

LAVENDER LOOSE PIGMENT

LIME GREEN EYE SHADOW

LIGHT SHIMMERY YELLOW GOLD LOOSE POWDER

COBALT BLUE GEL LINER

YELLOW GLITTER

CLEAR DUO

WATER

BLACK MASCARA

1 SET FLIRTY WISPIES STRIP LASHES

LONG INDIVIDUAL FLARE LASHES

BONE-COLORED EYE PENCIL

MAKEUP REMOVER

DEEP BRONZE GOLD MAKEUP

YELLOW GOLD MAKEUP

TRANSLUCENT POWDER

SHIMMERY CORAL BLUSH

BABY CORAL PINK LIP GLOSS

DEEP GOLD BODY MAKEUP

GOLD RAINBOW GLITTER

FOUNDATION BRUSHES

BEAUTYBLENDER

ANGLED EYEBROW BRUSH

EYE SHADOW BRUSHES

EYELINER BRUSH

CERAMIC BOWL

TISSUE

ROUNDED Q-TIPS

SMALL FAN BRUSH

SCOTCH TAPE

EYELASH CURLER

ORANGEWOOD STICK

POWDER BRUSH

BLUSH BRUSH

LIP BRUSH

BIG FLUFFY FAN BRUSH

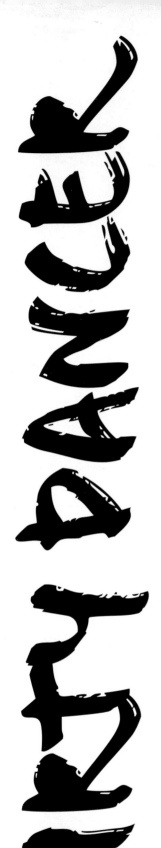

With all the tangos on *Dancing with the Stars*, there are only a few that stand out in my mind. Actress Jennifer Grey's was one of them. I was very excited to work with my *Dirty Dancing* starlet. She is a fiery sex pistol, funny, and witty. So here she is as a smoking-hot tango dancer. Perfect dancing makeup!

* Apply foundation to the eyes, up onto the forehead and into the hairline.

* With an angled eyebrow brush and clear wax with dark auburn eyebrow shadow, draw on dramatically arched eyebrows.

* Using an eye shadow brush, apply a matte gold cream eye shadow to the lid up to the crease in a big almond shape.

* Apply a steel gray cream eye shadow to the crease and above, getting higher onto the eye toward the outer corner, then rounded down to around the outer lower eye.

* With a gold loose pigment, go over the gold cream eye shadow to lock in the cream and intensify using a fluffy eye shadow brush.

* With a shimmery red brown eye shadow, go over the steel gray cream eye shadow to add dimension; blend.

* Use an eye shadow brush to apply a gray loose pigment over the crease, blending outward and then ending with a circular motion at the outer eye; blend well.

* Apply a black gel liner in a tight line all the way around the eye and then line the inner upper and lower waterlines, along with the inner tear duct, using an eyeliner brush.

* Apply foundation to the face, neck, and ears and down onto the chest.

* Apply a rose gold body makeup to the chest and shoulders; add a little to the upper cheekbones using a small foundation brush.

* Contour the nose, under the cheekbones and jawline, and in the décolletage with a gray/taupe cream contour color.

* Apply a peach cream blush to the cheeks.

* Blend this all in with foundation brushes and a Beautyblender.

* Powder the face with a light peach loose powder and powder puff.

* Line under the eye with gold loose pigment and a fat eyeliner brush.

* Curl the lashes and apply mascara. Apply a set of really big vampy strip lashes that are separated with triangular clumps, using dark Duo. Apply a set of big full plush strip lashes on top with dark Duo. Apply mascara again.

* Line the lips with a nude lip pencil. Apply a pinky nude lipstick and top off with a peach lip gloss.

TOOL KIT

FOUNDATION AND CONCEALER

CLEAR WAX AND DARK AUBURN EYEBROW SHADOW

MATTE GOLD CREAM EYE SHADOW

STEEL GRAY CREAM EYE SHADOW

GOLD LOOSE PIGMENT

SHIMMERY RED BROWN EYE SHADOW

GRAY LOOSE PIGMENT

BLACK GEL LINER

EYE MAKEUP REMOVER

ROSE GOLD BODY MAKEUP

GRAY/TAUPE CREAM CONTOUR COLOR

PEACH CREAM BLUSH

LIGHT PEACH LOOSE POWDER

BLACK MASCARA

1 SET BIG VAMPY STRIP LASHES WITH CLUMPS THAT ARE SEPARATED AND TRIANGULAR

1 SET BIG FULL PLUSH STRIP LASHES

DARK DUO

NUDE LIP PENCIL

PINKY NUDE LIPSTICK

PEACH LIP GLOSS

FOUNDATION BRUSHES

BEAUTYBLENDER

ANGLED EYEBROW BRUSH

EYE SHADOW BRUSHES

EYELINER BRUSHES

POWDER PUFF

POWDER BRUSH

EYELASH CURLER

SMALL FAN BRUSH

ORANGEWOOD STICK

LIP BRUSH

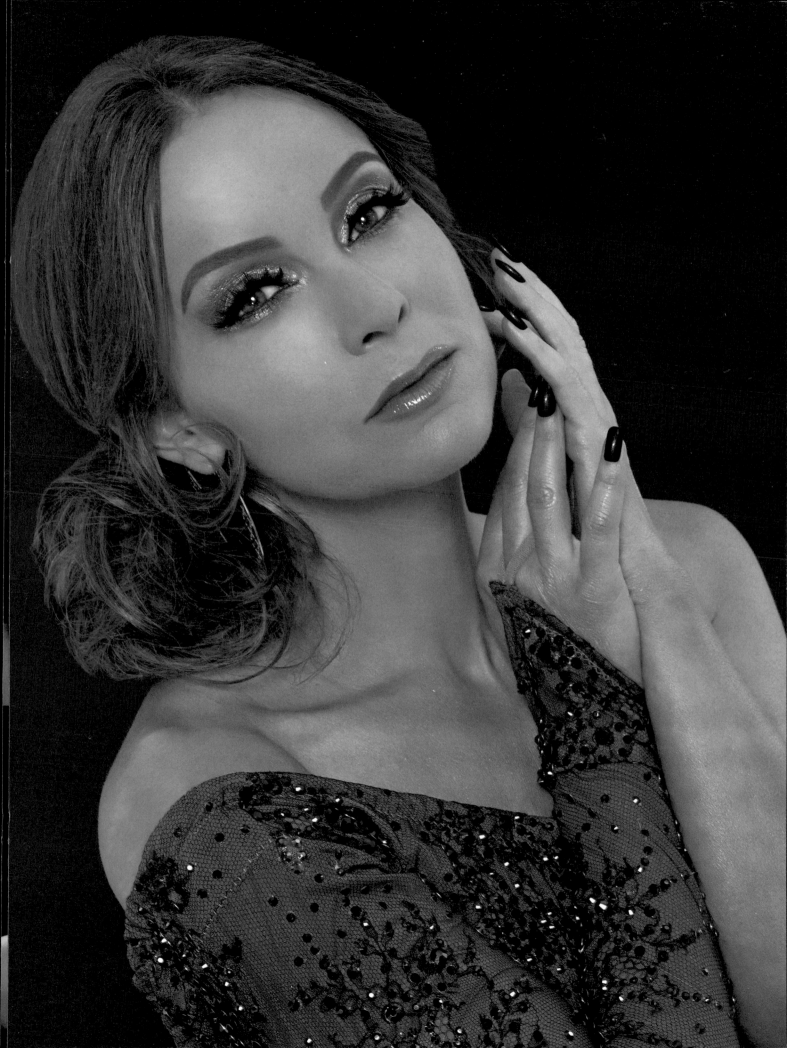

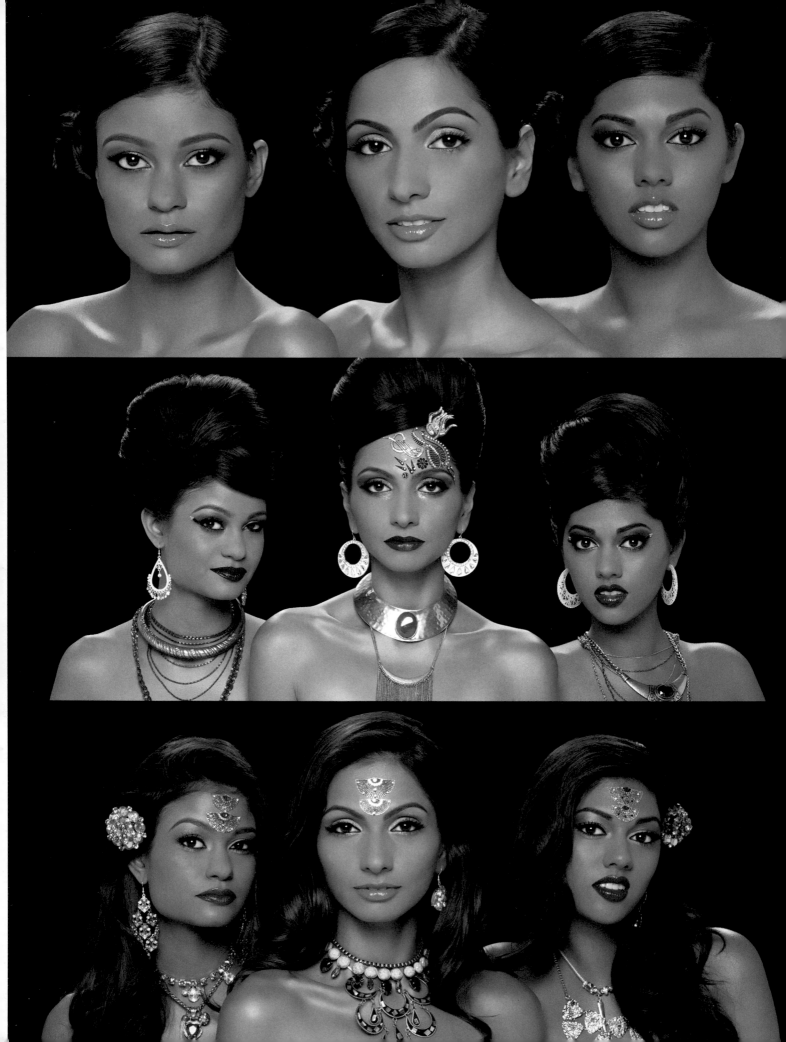

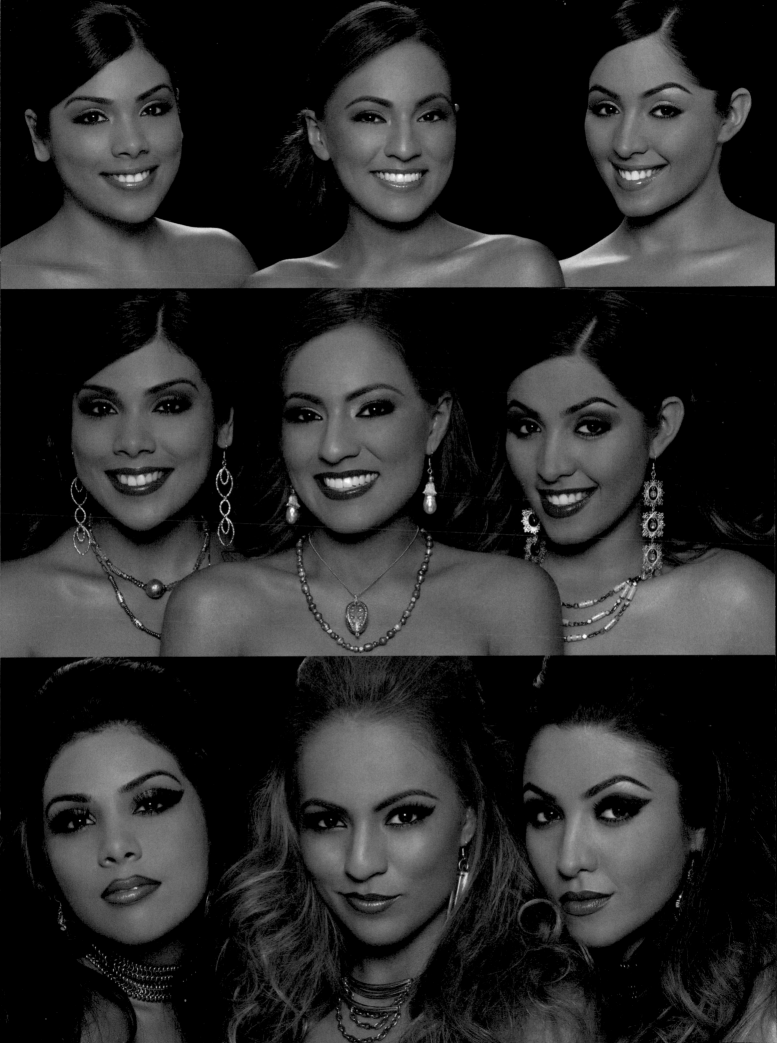

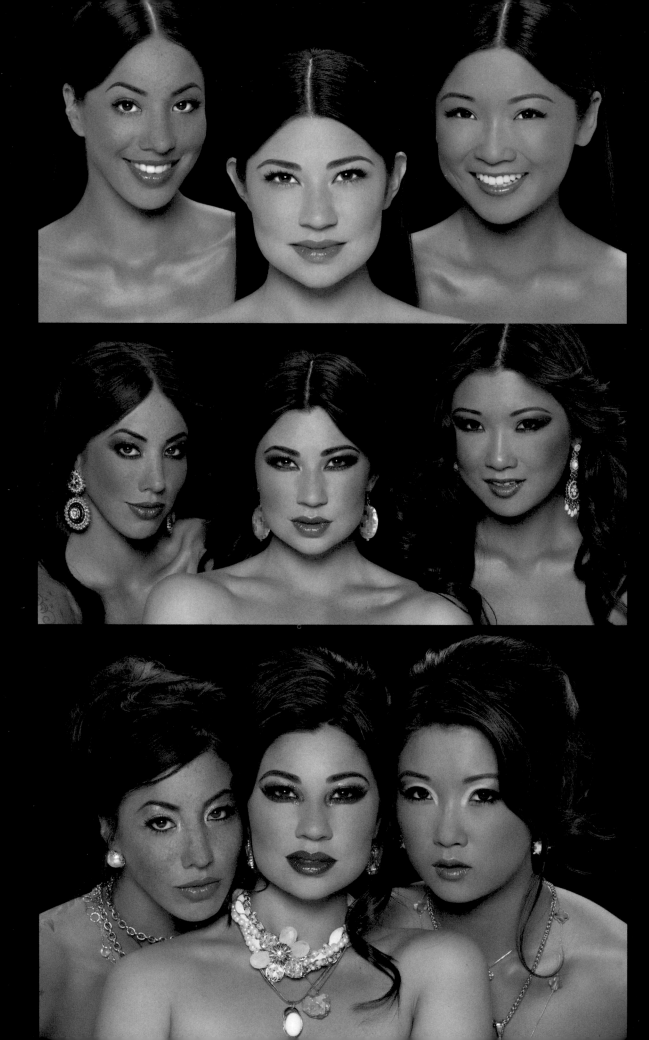

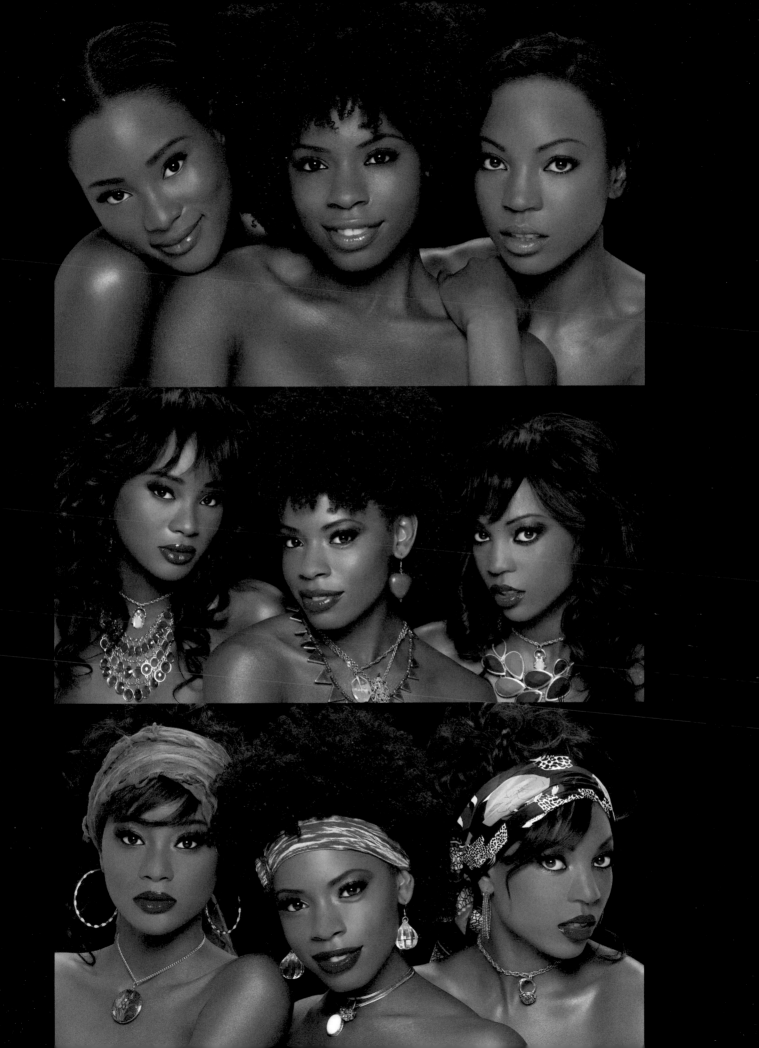

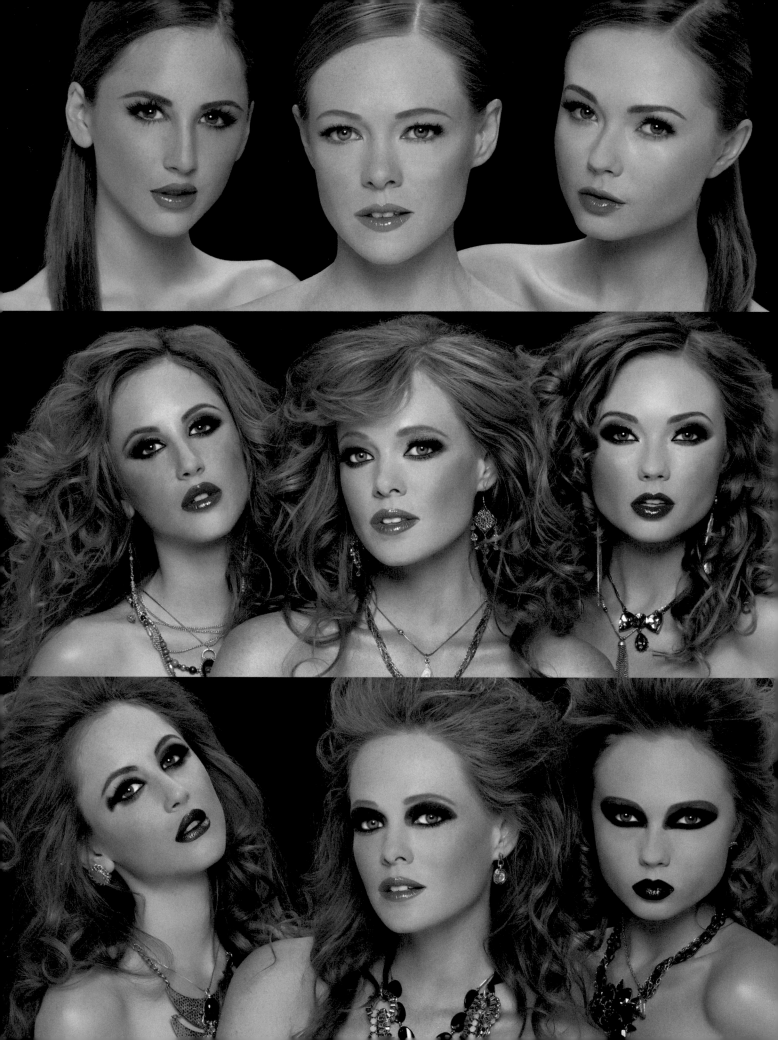

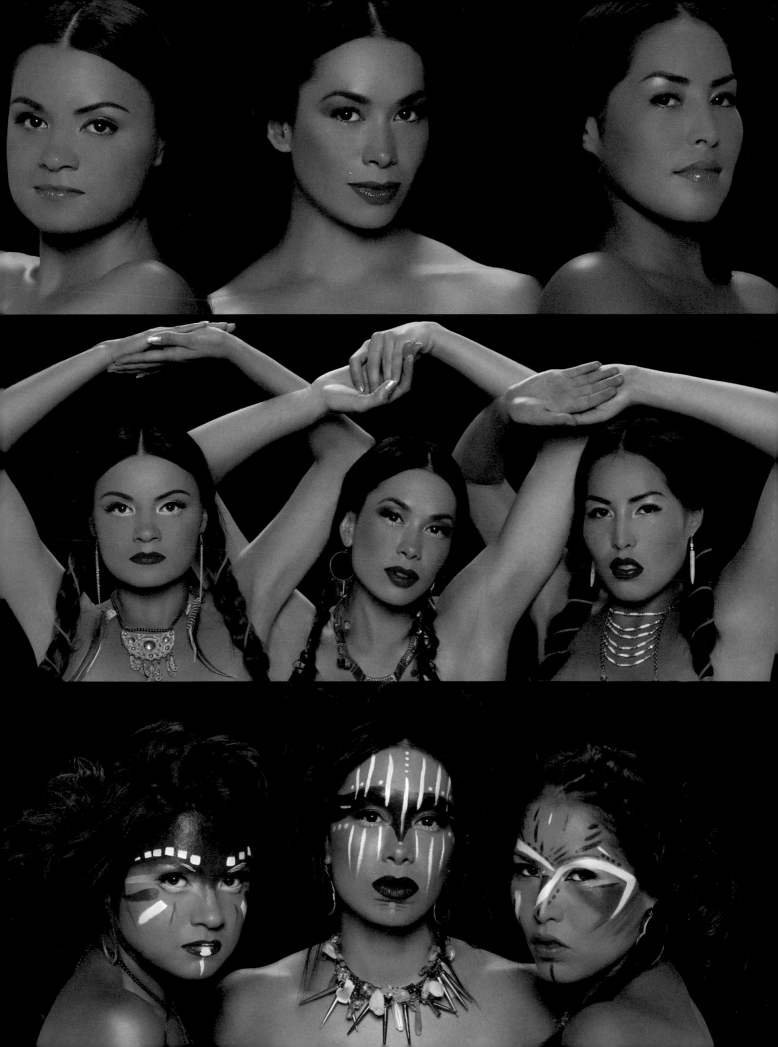

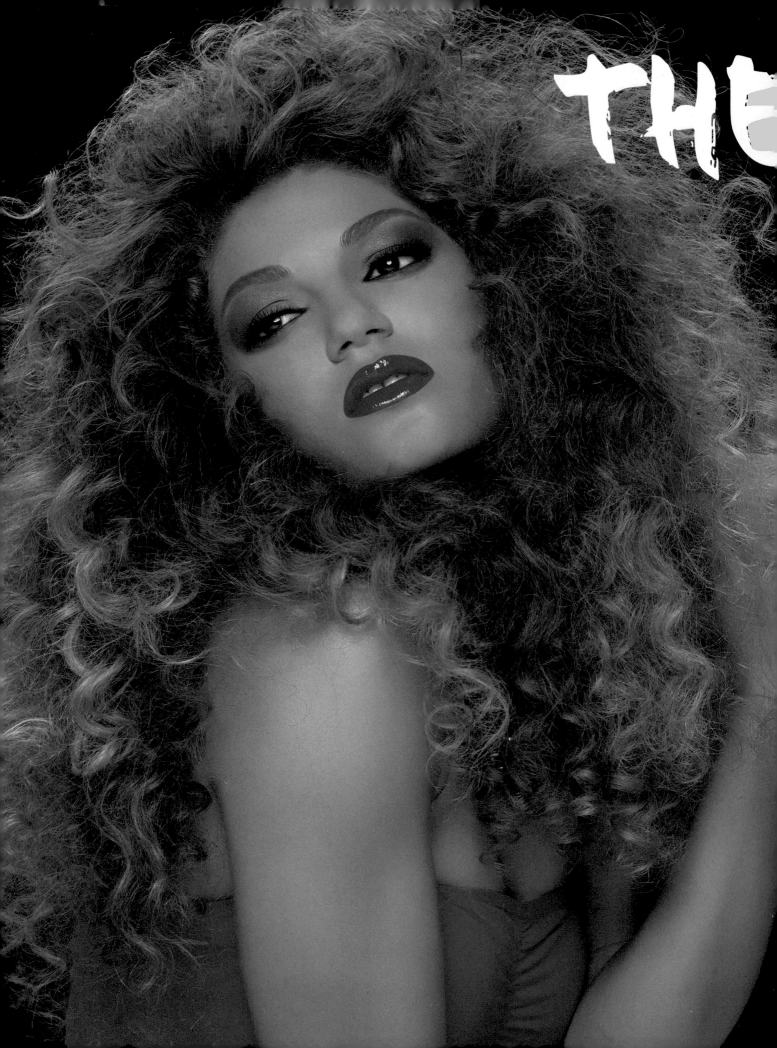

THE

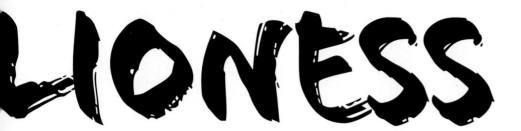

LIONESS

I love this Diana Ross–inspired makeup look. This is truly one of those looks that can be worn anywhere at anytime and is easy to achieve. This is timeless glamour. I love the brown shimmers mixed with light coppers and peachy golds. The red lip makes this look scream, "Kiss me!"

* Apply foundation to the face, eyes, neck, and ears.

* Contour down the sides of the nose and under the jawline with a medium brown cream contour color.

* Apply red cream blush to the apples of the cheeks.

* Add a rose gold makeup to foundation and apply on top of the red cream blush and under the lips in the center of the chin.

* Blend this all in with foundation brushes and a Beautyblender.

* Powder the T-zone with loose translucent powder.

* With a dark brown eyebrow pencil, draw in just at the top of the brow a defined line that tapers into a nice and precise brow end. With a smaller-than-usual angled eyebrow brush and medium brown eyebrow shadow, blend the pencil slightly.

* Using an eye shadow brush, apply a peachy gold eye shadow all over the eye, up to the brow, and around under the eye.

* Apply copper eye shadow all over the lid and then to the crease from the middle of the eye out toward the temple.

* Apply rich brown eye shadow to the outer crease and to the under crease.

* With a clean eye shadow brush, blend the brown into the crease and all colors seamlessly into each other, creating a beautiful fade.

* Line the inner upper and lower waterlines and around the inner tear duct with black gel liner. Tightly line the upper lash line.

* Curl the lashes and apply mascara.

* Apply two sets of full plush strip lashes that are different from each other to create texture using dark Duo.

* Apply mascara again.

* Apply a peachy bronzy shimmery blush to the cheeks with a fluffy blush brush.

* Line the lips with a cherry red lip liner.

* Apply an orange red lip gloss.

TOOL KIT

FOUNDATION AND CONCEALER

MEDIUM BROWN CONTOUR COLOR

RED CREAM BLUSH

ROSE GOLD MAKEUP

TRANSLUCENT POWDER

DARK BROWN EYEBROW PENCIL

MEDIUM BROWN EYEBROW SHADOW

PEACHY GOLD EYE SHADOW

COPPER EYE SHADOW

RICH BROWN EYE SHADOW

BLACK GEL LINER

BLACK MASCARA

2 SETS FULL PLUSH STRIP LASHES, EACH DIFFERENT

DARK DUO

PEACHY BRONZY SHIMMERY BLUSH

CHERRY RED LIP LINER

ORANGE RED LIP GLOSS

FOUNDATION BRUSHES

BEAUTYBLENDER

POWDER BRUSH

SMALLER-THAN-USUAL ANGLED EYEBROW BRUSH

EYE SHADOW BRUSHES

EYELINER BRUSHES

EYELASH CURLER

SMALL FAN BRUSH

ORANGEWOOD STICK

FLUFFY BLUSH BRUSH

LIP BRUSH

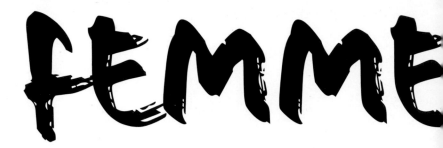

FEMME

When doing a photographic art installation for Concept L.A., I was looking for Asian models who were heavily and beautifully tattooed. Before the shoot I was still not able to cast the right girls, so I called local tattoo shops. This is how I learned about Kirsten. The next day she showed up to model, and we have been friends ever since. I love her freckles! I gave her sexy gray smoky eyes with browns, blacks, and apricots, along with bronzed skin. Blending cool and warm tones gives a special, dramatic effect.

* Apply foundation to the face, eyes, ears, and neck.

* Sculpt the cheeks, nose, and jawline with a bronze cream blush.

* Mix bronze cream blush with peach cream blush and apply to the cheekbones, blending up toward the temples.

* Add light gold makeup above and under the brow, on the tops of the cheeks, and under the lip.

* Apply a bronze gold makeup mixed with foundation all over the neck up to the jawline.

* Blend this all in with foundation brushes and a Beautyblender.

* Lightly dust the face with translucent powder and a fluffy powder brush.

* With an eye shadow brush, apply an apricot rust loose pigment on the lid, blending up and around the inner eye.

* Apply dark metallic gray eye shadow to create a gray smoke effect on the outer corners of the eyes; blend toward the lid and round around the outer edge and under the eye.

* Blend well in a circular motion with a clean brush.

* Apply brown cream eye shadow under the eye.

* With a short eyeliner brush, blend chocolate brown loose pigment under the whole eye and up to the outer corners.

* Use clear wax and dark brown eyebrow shadow with an angled eyebrow brush to draw a beautiful brow. Extend the brow end for added drama.

* Curl the lashes and apply mascara.

* Layer individual flare lashes in medium and long along the upper lash line, in a somewhat spacey manner, to create a flirty flare using dark Duo.

* Line the inner lower waterline with a copper eye pencil.

* With black gel liner, line the upper lash line with a very tight line.

* Apply mascara again.

* With a blush brush, add a hint of an orange blush high on the cheekbones.

* Use the copper eye pencil to fill in the lips.

* Apply rose gold lipstick to the lips.

* Dust deep bronze loose powder with a fluffy blush brush to the cheeks and shoulders.

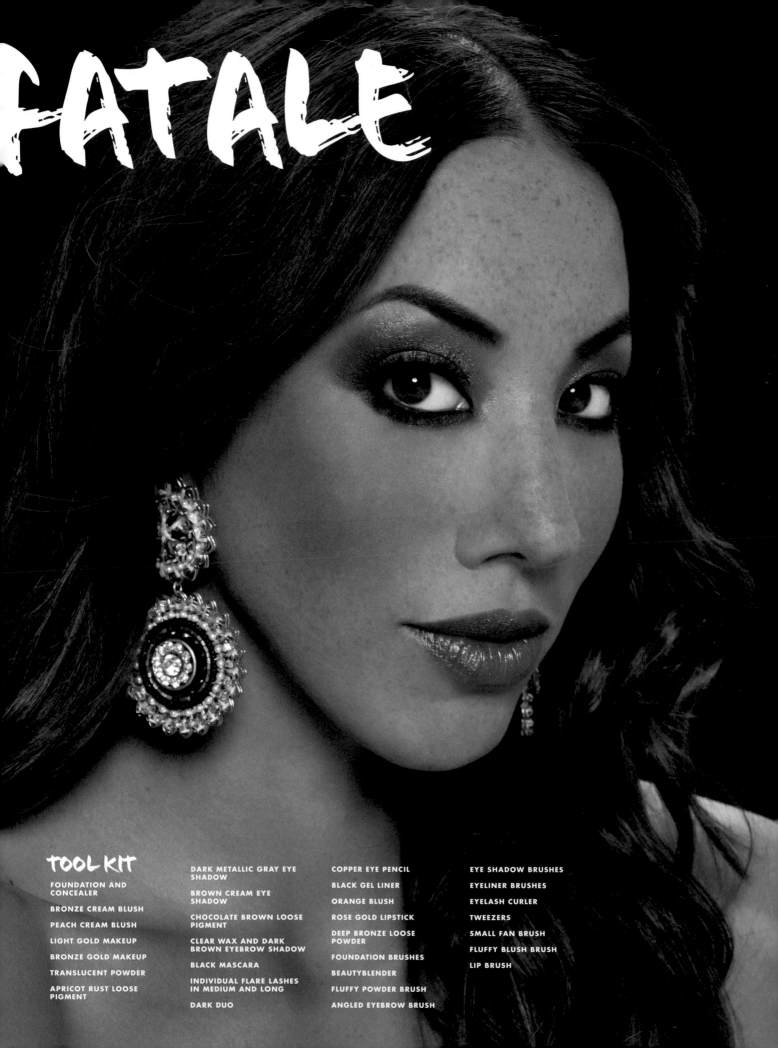

FATALE

TOOL KIT

FOUNDATION AND
CONCEALER

BRONZE CREAM BLUSH

PEACH CREAM BLUSH

LIGHT GOLD MAKEUP

BRONZE GOLD MAKEUP

TRANSLUCENT POWDER

APRICOT RUST LOOSE
PIGMENT

DARK METALLIC GRAY EYE
SHADOW

BROWN CREAM EYE
SHADOW

CHOCOLATE BROWN LOOSE
PIGMENT

CLEAR WAX AND DARK
BROWN EYEBROW SHADOW

BLACK MASCARA

INDIVIDUAL FLARE LASHES
IN MEDIUM AND LONG

DARK DUO

COPPER EYE PENCIL

BLACK GEL LINER

ORANGE BLUSH

ROSE GOLD LIPSTICK

DEEP BRONZE LOOSE
POWDER

FOUNDATION BRUSHES

BEAUTYBLENDER

FLUFFY POWDER BRUSH

ANGLED EYEBROW BRUSH

EYE SHADOW BRUSHES

EYELINER BRUSHES

EYELASH CURLER

TWEEZERS

SMALL FAN BRUSH

FLUFFY BLUSH BRUSH

LIP BRUSH

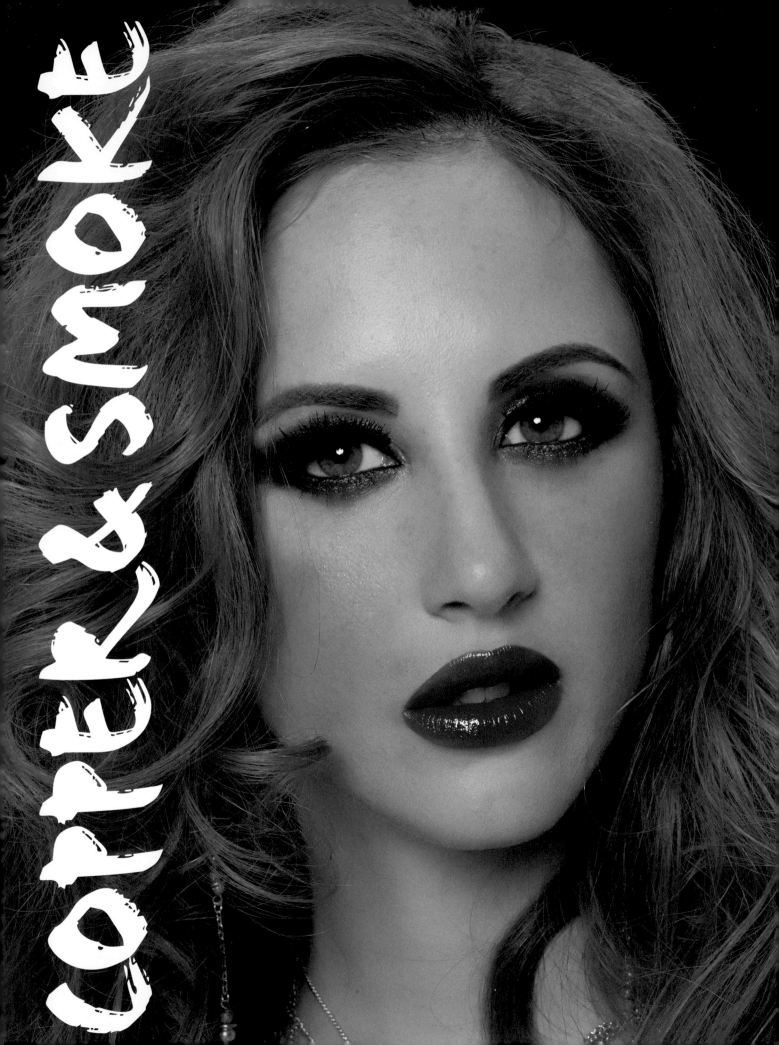

copper & smoke

I love having Faith at my Gleam shoots. She is super professional, positive, and also a lot of fun. It's been great to watch her career flourish. When making up redheads, I am instantly drawn to browns, rusts, coppers, and blacks. For this look, I wanted to create sophisticated glamour with a smoky eye.

✴ Apply foundation over the eyes and up to the forehead.

✴ Use a thin red eyebrow pencil to draw in the eyebrow shape, round the arch, and extend up and out.

✴ Using an angled eyebrow brush, go over the pencil to soften a bit with an auburn red eyebrow shadow.

✴ With an eye shadow brush, apply brown cream eye shadow to the crease and above, connecting the outer undereye, and blend.

✴ Apply a copper cream eye shadow all over the lid.

✴ Lock in the cream on the lid with copper reflects loose powder using an eye shadow brush.

✴ With a thin eye shadow brush, apply chocolate brown eye shadow, blending into the crease and toward the outer eye, extending the eye to make it look bigger and almond shaped, and then round down under the outer corner of the eye.

✴ Clean up under the brow with foundation.

✴ With a small fluffy eye shadow brush, apply a light yellow gold loose powder around the tear duct in a circular motion and add just a bit under the corner of the eye.

✴ Line the inner upper and lower waterlines with black gel liner; also line the upper lash line with a cat line, using a pointy eyeliner brush.

✴ Curl the lashes and apply mascara.

✴ Apply the copper loose powder again under the eye to the center and let it fall a bit.

✴ Clean up under the eyes with makeup remover.

✴ Apply one set of Andrea Modlash #33s with dark Duo.

✴ Lay individual flare lashes in short, medium, and long into the strip lashes with dark Duo.

✴ Go over the upper liner with another coat of black gel liner.

✴ Apply mascara again.

✴ Apply foundation to the rest of the face, ears, and neck.

✴ Apply a bronze copper cream blush to the cheeks with a foundation brush.

✴ Blend this all in with foundation brushes and a Beautyblender.

✴ Lightly dust the face with translucent powder and a fluffy powder brush.

✴ Apply a bright coral shimmery blush to the apples of the cheeks and blend up toward the temple.

✴ Line and fill in the lips with a brown lip pencil.

✴ Apply a brick-red lip gloss on top.

TOOL KIT

FOUNDATION AND CONCEALER

THIN RED EYEBROW PENCIL

AUBURN RED EYEBROW SHADOW

BROWN CREAM EYE SHADOW

COPPER CREAM EYE SHADOW

COPPER REFLECTS LOOSE POWDER

CHOCOLATE BROWN EYE SHADOW

LIGHT YELLOW GOLD LOOSE POWDER

BLACK GEL LINER

BLACK MASCARA

EYE MAKEUP REMOVER

1 SET ANDREA MODLASH #33S

INDIVIDUAL FLARE LASHES IN SHORT, MEDIUM, AND LONG

DARK DUO

BRONZE COPPER CREAM BLUSH

TRANSLUCENT POWDER

BRIGHT CORAL SHIMMERY BLUSH

BROWN LIP PENCIL

BRICK-RED LIP GLOSS

FOUNDATION BRUSHES

BEAUTYBLENDER

ANGLED EYEBROW BRUSH

EYE SHADOW BRUSHES

EYELINER BRUSHES

EYELASH CURLER

ORANGEWOOD STICK

TWEEZERS

BLUSH BRUSH

FLUFFY POWDER BRUSH

LIP BRUSH

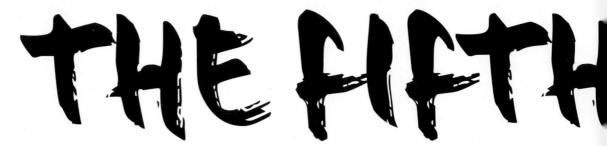

THE FIFTH

When we spoke of Chandon's home, I remembered Bollywood films depicting extravagant, luscious celebrations, with rich colors everywhere. I imagined rich chocolates, rusts, and golds, along with bindis and jewels to add sparkle.

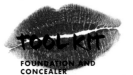

TOOL KIT

FOUNDATION AND CONCEALER

TRANSLUCENT POWDER

CLEAR WAX AND DARK BROWN EYEBROW SHADOW

SHIMMERY APRICOT GOLD LOOSE PIGMENT

CHOCOLATE BROWN LOOSE PIGMENT

YELLOW GOLD EYE SHADOW

BLACK GEL LINER

SHIMMERY RICH RUSTY BROWN EYE SHADOW

BLACK MASCARA

2 SETS WISPIES STRIP LASHES

DARK AND CLEAR DUO

EYE MAKEUP REMOVER

ROSE GOLD MAKEUP

GRAY/TAUPE CREAM CONTOUR COLOR

CRANBERRY MATTE BLUSH

DARK CRANBERRY LIP LINER

DARK CRANBERRY LIPSTICK

BODY ART, BINDIS, AND RHINESTONES

FOUNDATION BRUSHES

BEAUTYBLENDER

POWDER BRUSH

ANGLED EYEBROW BRUSH

EYE SHADOW BRUSHES

EYELINER BRUSHES

EYELASH CURLER

ORANGEWOOD STICK

LATEX SPONGES

CONTOURED BLUSH BRUSH

LIP BRUSH

* Apply foundation all over the eyelids and up to the forehead.

* Lightly powder.

* With an angled eyebrow brush, intensify the eyebrows with clear wax and dark brown eyebrow shadow.

* Apply a shimmery apricot gold loose pigment to the eyelids.

* With a skinny eye shadow brush, apply chocolate brown loose pigment to the crease and extend out as far as the end of the brow. Take the brown almost all the way up to the brow, leaving just a small space under the brow, then blend to the outer crease, connecting the brown under the eye. Blend well.

* With a small shadow brush, apply yellow gold eye shadow in a circular motion to the inner eye around the tear duct; line under the eye and stop at the middle.

* Use a small foundation brush and a little of the foundation to clean up under the brow.

* Line the inner upper and lower waterlines. With a black gel liner, also line the inner tear duct. Line the upper lash line with a tight line.

* Soften the upper liner by blending a shimmery rich rusty brown eye shadow on top, using an eyeliner brush.

* Curl the lashes and apply mascara.

* Apply two sets of Wispies strip lashes using dark Duo.

* With makeup remover and a latex sponge, clean up under the eye.

* Apply foundation to the rest of the face, ears, and neck.

* Mix a rose gold makeup into foundation and apply to the cheeks.

* Contour by painting lines down the sides of nose, under the cheekbones, and heavily along the jawline using a gray/taupe cream contour color.

* Blend this all in with foundation brushes and a Beautyblender.

* Lightly powder the face with translucent powder.

* Sweep a cranberry matte blush onto the high part of the cheekbones, using a contoured blush brush.

* Line the lips and fill in with a dark cranberry lip liner. Apply a dark cranberry lipstick with a touch of sheen.

* The fun part of this look is adding the body art and bindis. Find and choose some Sumita body art from Ziba Beauty and a few clear Swarovski crystals. Most brands have glue on the back, but to ensure they stick properly, give an extra bit of staying power by brushing some clear Duo onto the back. Let the pieces get tacky, then lay them down and be artistic.

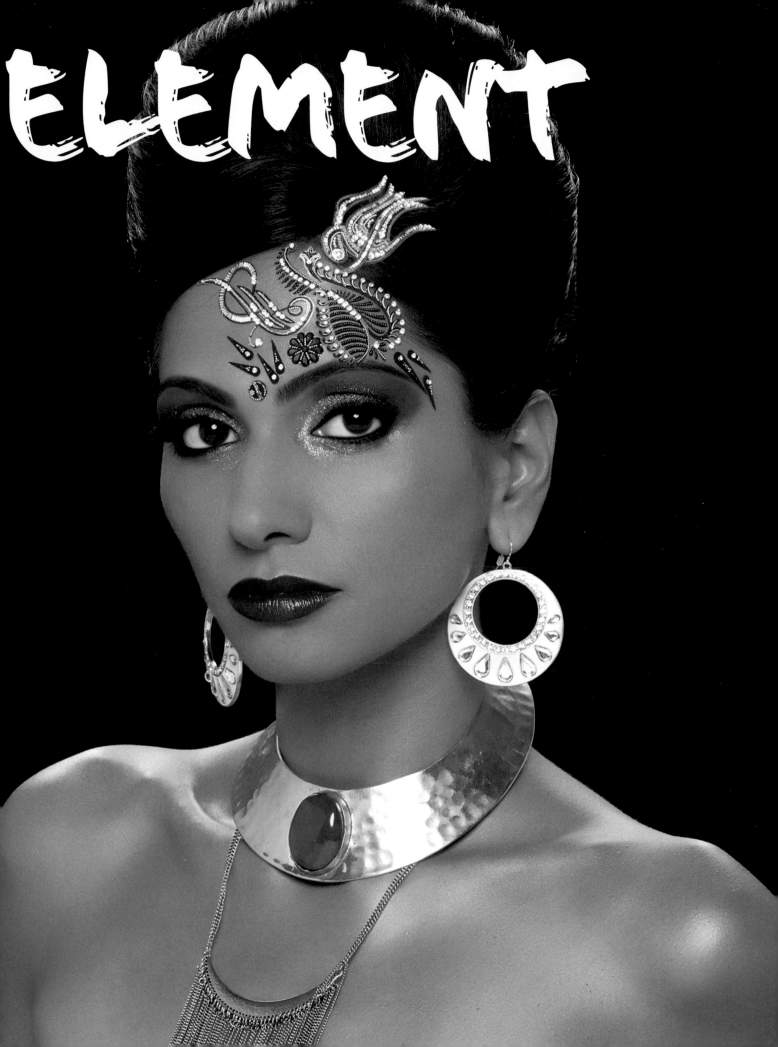

ELEMENT

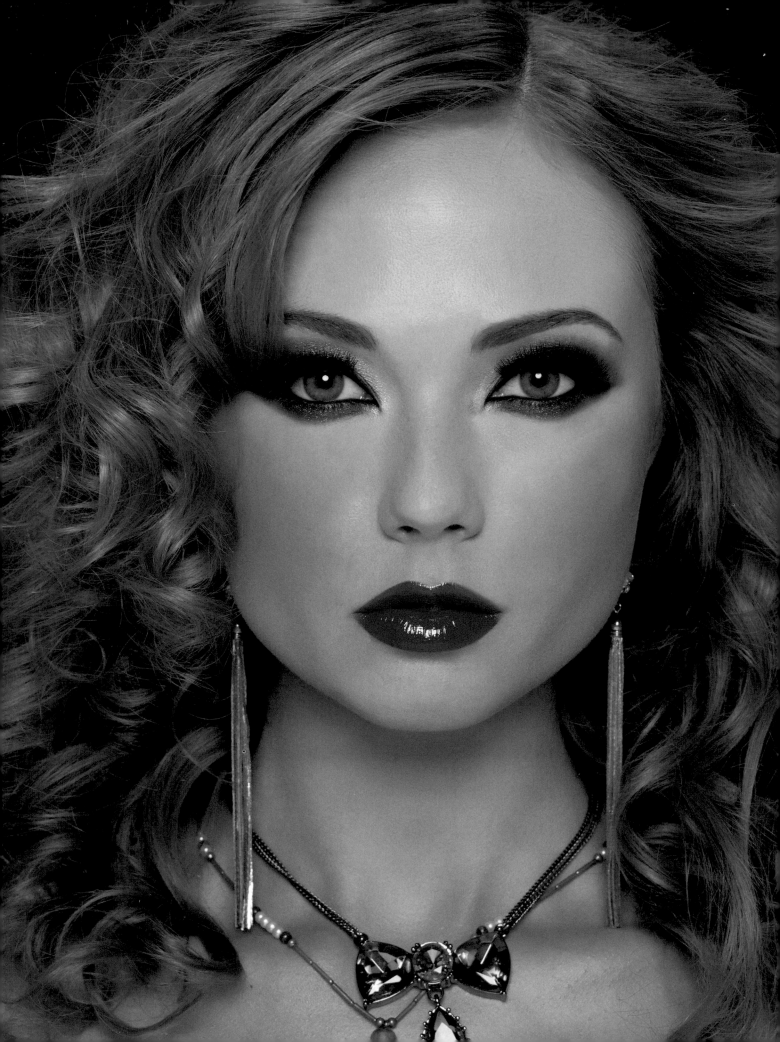

Marketa's look epitomizes sexy yet sophisticated. It's a modern smoky eye. The makeup gives her a lit-from-within glow that screams, "Look at my gorgeous face!" While the colors are complementary to her coloring, you'll find that anyone can wear shades of copper with accents of black and yellow and look stunning. This look was chosen for the cover because it's full of gleam, glitter, and glam and is one that anyone can achieve.

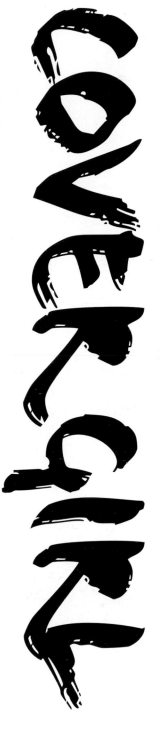

* Apply foundation to the eyes and forehead and into the hairline.

* Draw in the brows using an angled eyebrow brush with clear wax and auburn red eyebrow shadow. I kept them pretty natural with an extra touch of definition.

* With a small eye shadow brush, apply shimmery red brown loose pigment to the lid up to the crease toward the outer eye a little past the end of the brow, then back down at a strong angle under all of the eye thickly.

* Using a small crease eye shadow brush, apply a glittery copper loose pigment to the middle of the eyelid up on and above the crease, blending back toward the inner eye. Apply only to the middle of under the eye and blend back and forth; let it fall.

* With a small eye shadow brush, apply shimmery yellow eye shadow to the inner eye and around the tear duct, blending into other colors.

* Clean up under the eyes with makeup remover. Use the edge of the latex sponge with a little remover to cut a hard line for under the shadow liner.

* Apply foundation to the rest of the face, neck, and ears.

* Apply rose gold body makeup all over the chest and up the neckline; apply a little to the upper cheekbones.

* Contour down the sides of the nose and under the cheekbones down toward the lips at an angle with a gray/taupe cream contour color.

* Apply peach cream blush.

* Blend this all in with foundation brushes and a Beautyblender.

* Lightly powder the face with translucent powder and a powder brush.

* Line the inner upper and lower waterlines with black gel liner along with a tight line to the upper lash line.

* Curl the lashes and apply mascara.

* Apply one set of Wispies strip lashes with dark Duo.

* Lay individual flare lashes in medium and long into the outer lash line within the strip lash using dark Duo.

* Apply mascara again.

* Use a blush brush to apply a sparkly orange blush to the cheeks.

* Line and fill in the lips with a deep red lip liner.

* Apply a brick-red lip gloss.

TOOL KIT

FOUNDATION AND CONCEALER	**SHIMMERY YELLOW EYE SHADOW**	**BLACK MASCARA**	**FOUNDATION BRUSHES**	**SMALL FAN BRUSH**
CLEAR WAX AND AUBURN RED EYEBROW SHADOW	**EYE MAKEUP REMOVER**	**1 SET WISPIES STRIP LASHES**	**BEAUTYBLENDER**	**ORANGEWOOD STICK**
SHIMMERY RED BROWN LOOSE PIGMENT	**ROSE GOLD BODY MAKEUP**	**INDIVIDUAL FLARE LASHES IN MEDIUM AND LONG**	**ANGLED EYEBROW BRUSH**	**TWEEZERS**
GLITTERY COPPER LOOSE PIGMENT	**GRAY/TAUPE CREAM CONTOUR COLOR**	**DARK DUO**	**EYE SHADOW BRUSHES**	**BLUSH BRUSH**
	PEACH CREAM BLUSH	**SPARKLY ORANGE BLUSH**	**LATEX SPONGE**	**LIP BRUSH**
	TRANSLUCENT POWDER	**DEEP RED LIP LINER**	**POWDER BRUSH**	
	BLACK GEL LINER	**BRICK-RED LIP GLOSS**	**EYELINER BRUSHES**	
			EYELASH CURLER	

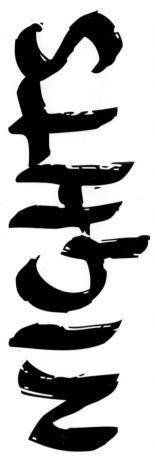

TOKYO NIGHTS

I have always been drawn to peacock colors and neons. When I was young I swore to my mom that my best friend, Lori, and I would bring back neon. Well, neon is back, but it just happened again like all the other eras of makeup and style. This look was inspired by a Neo Tokyo girl pop band and pictures of the neon lights that stud Tokyo's nightlife.

* Apply foundation to the eyes and forehead and into the hairline.

* With a dark brown eyebrow pencil, draw in eyebrows. I kept them natural.

* Use an angled eyebrow brush with clear wax and dark brown eyebrow shadow on top of the brow liner to soften.

* The next three steps use cream eye shadow and various sizes of eye shadow brushes and eyeliner brushes.

* Apply a bright green cream eye shadow under all of the eye and around the tear duct toward the lid.

* Apply a neon lime green cream shadow on top of the green to the upper tear duct area; thickly paint upward toward the brow and toward the upper crease.

* Apply a neon blue cream eye shadow on top of the lime green from the middle of the crease to the outer corner of the eye; draw that line straight to create an angled edge, then come back down in a triangle shape to the outer undereye.

* With a short blunt eyeliner brush, blend the edges of color into one another.

* Apply a little foundation under the brow to keep a clean space.

* Blend translucent powder over the eye makeup, locking in the creams while slightly blending.

* Clean up under the eyes with the edge of a latex sponge and gel eye makeup remover and sweep out toward the eye.

* Apply foundation to the rest of the face, neck, and ears.

* Apply a soft baby pink cream blush to the apples of the cheeks.

* Blend this all in with foundation brushes and a Beautyblender.

* Powder the face with translucent powder and a powder puff, brushing off any excess with a powder brush.

* Line the inner upper and lower waterlines and the inner tear duct with black gel liner.

* Curl the lashes and apply mascara.

* Apply individual flare lashes in short, medium, and long to the lash line with dark Duo.

* Apply mascara again.

* Apply shimmery pink blush to the cheeks with a blush brush.

* Line the lips with a brown nude lip pencil.

* Apply a shimmery light pink lipstick.

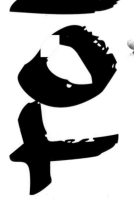

TOOL KIT

FOUNDATION AND CONCEALER

DARK BROWN EYEBROW PENCIL

CLEAR WAX AND DARK BROWN EYEBROW SHADOW

BRIGHT GREEN, NEON LIME GREEN, AND NEON BLUE CREAM EYE SHADOWS

TRANSLUCENT POWDER

GEL EYE MAKEUP REMOVER

SOFT BABY PINK CREAM BLUSH

BLACK GEL LINER

BLACK MASCARA

INDIVIDUAL FLARE LASHES IN SHORT, MEDIUM, AND LONG

DARK DUO

SHIMMERY PINK BLUSH

BROWN NUDE LIP PENCIL

SHIMMERY LIGHT PINK LIPSTICK

FOUNDATION BRUSHES

BEAUTYBLENDER

EYE SHADOW BRUSHES

EYELINER BRUSHES

LATEX SPONGE

POWDER PUFF

POWDER BRUSH

LATEX SPONGE

EYELASH CURLER

SMALL FAN BRUSH

TWEEZERS

BLUSH BRUSH

LIP BRUSH

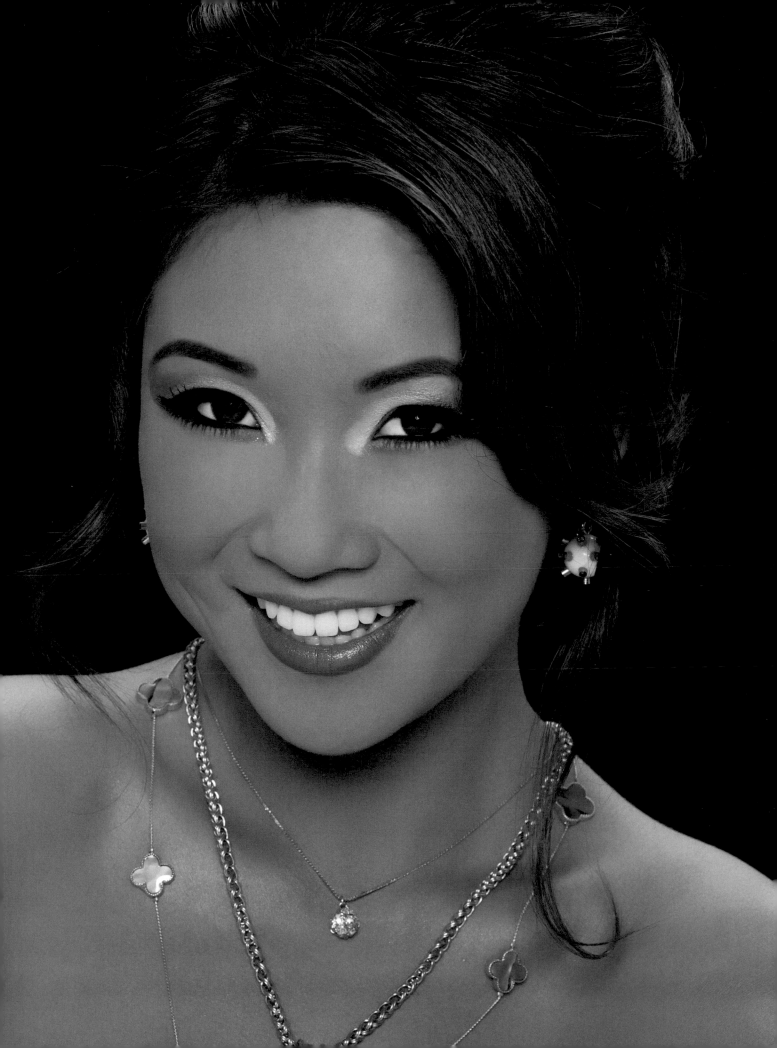

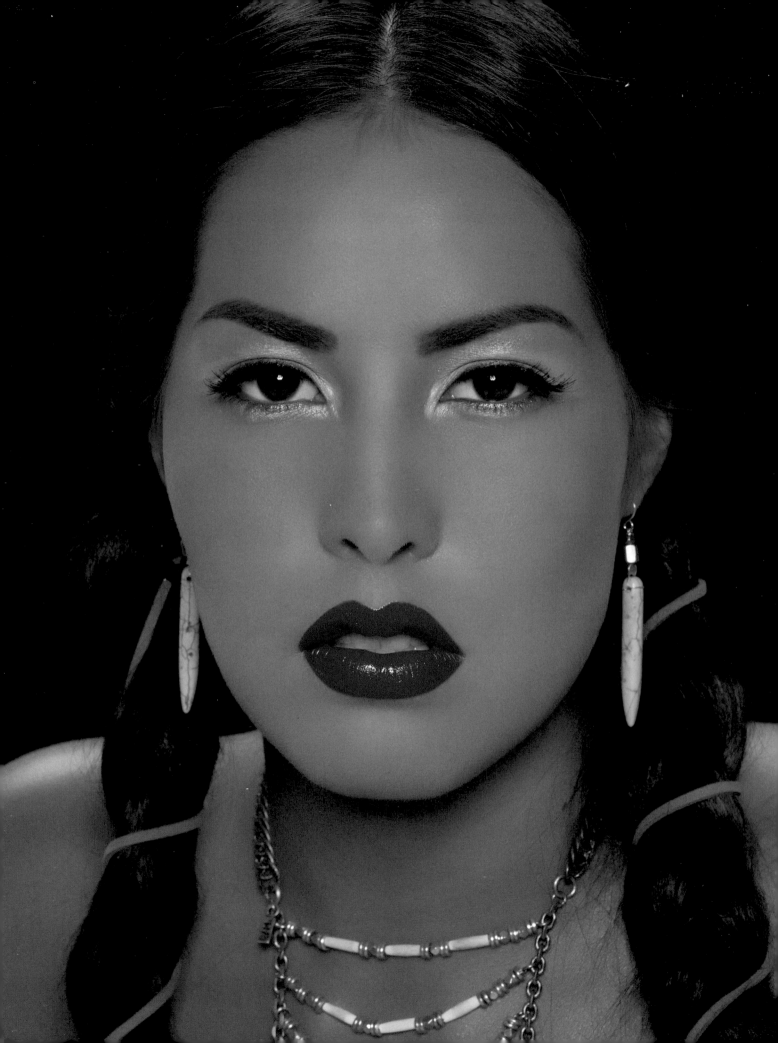

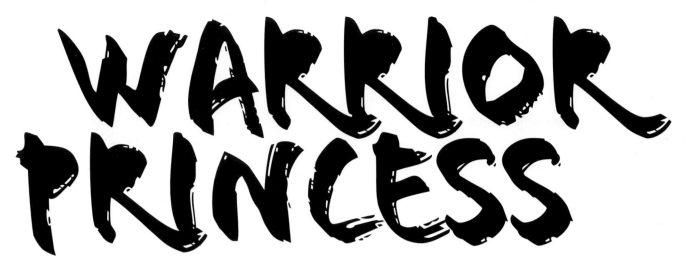

WARRIOR PRINCESS

This makeup wows in its simplicity. Using a creamy turquoise shimmer with an even gold complexion and a solid red lip is pure Americana at its best.

* Apply foundation to the face, eyes, neck, and ears and up into the hairline.

* Contour under the cheekbones starting at the hollows near the temple and under the jawline using a gray/taupe cream contour color.

* Apply red cream blush to the cheeks.

* Blend this all in with foundation brushes and a Beautyblender.

* Powder the face with translucent powder and a powder brush.

* Using an angled eyebrow brush with clear wax and dark brown eyebrow shadow, fill in the brows naturally.

* With an eye shadow brush, apply a shimmery green eye shadow to the lids and up to and above the crease around the inner eye down on top of the tear duct; blend well.

* Apply a shimmery baby blue eye shadow all under the eye, connecting with the green at both the tear duct and the outer eye. With the same blue, lightly sweep over the green on the lid.

* Apply black gel liner to the inner upper and lower waterlines and around the inner tear duct, then tightly line the upper lash line using a pointy eyeliner brush.

* Curl the lashes and apply mascara.

* Lay in individual flare lashes in short, medium, and long with dark Duo.

* Apply mascara again.

* Apply a matte red blush to the cheeks with a blush brush.

* Line and fill in the lips with a cranberry lip pencil.

* Apply a cherry red lipstick.

* Apply a rose gold body makeup to the chest and up the neckline.

TOOL KIT

FOUNDATION AND CONCEALER	SHIMMERY GREEN EYE SHADOW	DARK DUO	POWDER BRUSH	BLUSH BRUSH
GRAY/TAUPE CREAM CONTOUR COLOR	SHIMMERY BABY BLUE EYE SHADOW	MATTE RED BLUSH	ANGLED EYEBROW BRUSH	LIP BRUSH
RED CREAM BLUSH	BLACK GEL LINER	CRANBERRY LIP PENCIL	EYE SHADOW BRUSHES	
TRANSLUCENT POWDER	BLACK MASCARA	CHERRY RED LIPSTICK	EYELINER BRUSHES	
CLEAR WAX AND DARK BROWN EYEBROW SHADOW	INDIVIDUAL FLARE LASHES IN SHORT, MEDIUM, AND LONG	ROSE GOLD BODY MAKEUP	EYELASH CURLER	
		FOUNDATION BRUSHES	SMALL FAN BRUSH	
		BEAUTYBLENDER	TWEEZERS	

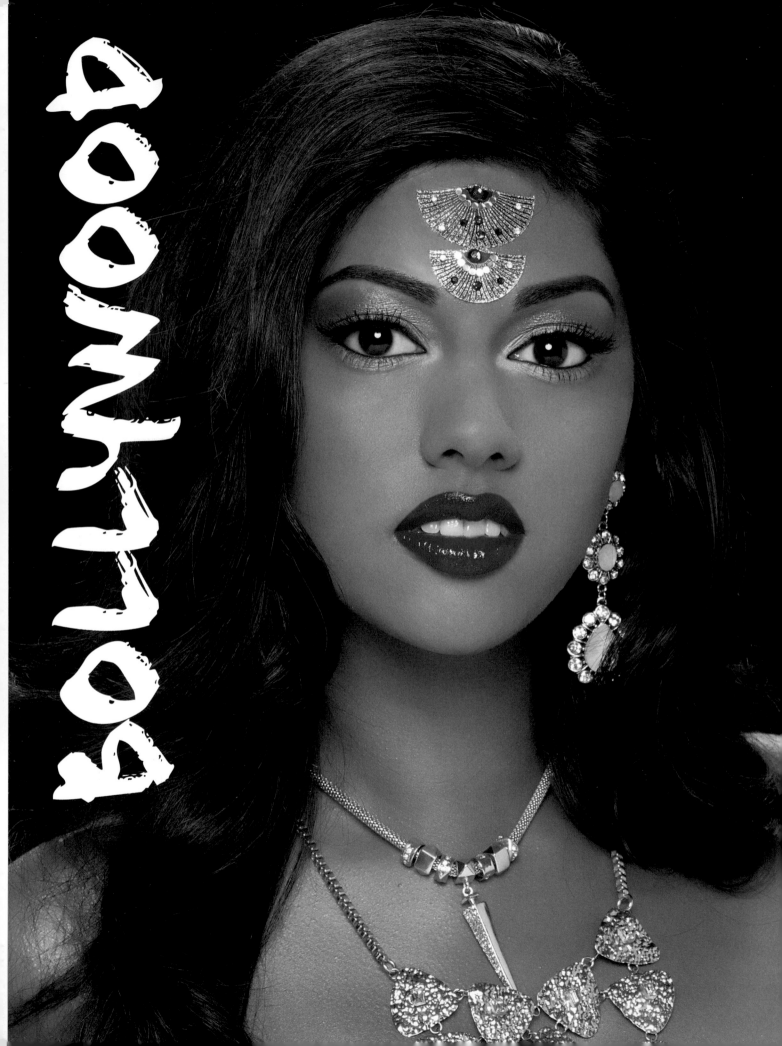

Sheena was another wonderful referral through Facebook. She is an exquisite East Indian beauty, and her look was inspired by colorful Indian weddings. I love Bollywood films where everybody is wrapped in rich, bright, beautiful silks and the streets are decked out with flowers and colorful flags. The women in these movies always have beautiful kohl-lined eyes. All shades of greens are amazing on Sheena's skin tone. This is a fun makeup look for shopping at the mall with friends or that Saturday night party.

* Apply foundation to the eyes and forehead, blending into the hairline.

* Apply an olive eye shadow with a touch of gold to the lid and blend in with a regular eye shadow brush.

* With a thin eye shadow brush, apply a teal blue eye shadow to the crease and around the outer edge of the eye in a round motion.

* Use a small fluffy eyeliner brush to apply a kelly green eye shadow under the eye, starting at the tear duct and then connecting to the outer eye and blending into the teal blue. Blend well.

* With a small foundation brush and a touch of foundation, clean up under the brow.

* Using a clear wax with dark brown eyebrow shadow, fill in the eyebrows using an angled eyebrow brush.

* Line the inner upper and lower waterlines and inner tear duct using black gel liner and a pointy eyeliner brush. Line the upper lash line very precisely and tightly all the way around the tear duct as well.

* Curl the lashes and apply mascara.

* Apply one set of Demi Wispies strip lashes using dark Duo.

* Lay in individual flare lashes in short, medium, and long with dark Duo, and fill in along the upper lash line on top of the Demi Wispies.

* Apply mascara again.

* Clean up under the eyes with makeup remover.

* Apply foundation to the rest of the face, neck, and ears.

* Contour along the jawline with an almond brown cream contour color.

* Apply red cream blush to the cheeks.

* Blend this all in with foundation brushes and a Beautyblender.

* Dust the face with translucent powder.

* Apply baby pink matte blush with a fluffy blush brush to the apples of the cheeks and sweep up to the outer corner of the eye.

* Use Sumita body art from Ziba for a dramatic bindi art. Paint the back of the jewel piece with clear Duo, let it get tacky for a few seconds, and then apply.

* Add individual Swarovski crystals around the bindis to enhance.

* Line and fill in the lips with a cranberry lip pencil.

* Apply a hot pink lip gloss.

TOOL KIT

FOUNDATION AND CONCEALER

OLIVE GOLD EYE SHADOW

TEAL BLUE EYE SHADOW

KELLY GREEN EYE SHADOW

CLEAR WAX AND DARK BROWN EYEBROW SHADOW

BLACK GEL LINER

BLACK MASCARA

1 SET DEMI WISPIES STRIP LASHES

INDIVIDUAL FLARE LASHES IN SHORT, MEDIUM, AND LONG

DARK AND CLEAR DUO

MAKEUP REMOVER

ALMOND BROWN CREAM CONTOUR COLOR

RED CREAM BLUSH

TRANSLUCENT POWDER

BABY PINK MATTE BLUSH

BINDI BODY AND FACE ART

SWAROVSKI CRYSTALS

CRANBERRY LIP PENCIL

HOT PINK LIP GLOSS

FOUNDATION BRUSHES

BEAUTYBLENDER

EYE SHADOW BRUSHES

ANGLED EYEBROW BRUSH

EYELINER BRUSHES

EYELASH CURLER

SMALL FAN BRUSH

ORANGEWOOD STICK

TWEEZERS

POWDER BRUSH

FLUFFY BLUSH BRUSH

LIP BRUSH

TEQUILA SUNRISE

I wanted to include makeup that reminded me of one of my favorite places in the world: Mexico, with its exotic bright yellows, oranges, fuchsia pinks, and reds. Here's a glamorous look that will be sure to grab attention. Stand out in the crowd!

* Apply foundation to over the eyes and up onto the forehead and into the hairline.

* With an eye shadow brush, apply a bright orange loose pigment to the lid.

* Apply a yellow gold eye shadow under the eye and around the tear duct; blend in with a small eye shadow brush.

* Apply an electric red orange loose pigment to the crease and above with a small eye shadow brush; blend well.

* Blend a pinky champagne eye shadow under the brow bone.

* Brush out the brows and use a dark brown eyebrow pencil to draw in an extreme rounded arch.

* Soften by applying dark brown eyebrow shadow to the brow and extend the brow end.

* Clean up under the eyes with makeup remover.

* Apply foundation to the rest of the face, neck, and ears.

* Apply orange peach cream blush.

* Blend this all in with foundation brushes and a Beautyblender.

* Apply black gel liner to the inner and upper waterlines and inner tear duct; also line all the way around the eye, thicker at the outer corners.

* Curl the lashes and apply mascara.

* Apply one set of big plush strip lashes with dark Duo.

* Apply mascara again.

* Lightly powder the face with a light peach loose powder.

* Apply a shimmery coral peach blush to the cheeks.

* Line the lips with a hot pink lip liner.

* Top off the lips with a hot pink lip gloss.

TOOL KIT

FOUNDATION AND CONCEALER

ORANGE LOOSE PIGMENT

YELLOW GOLD EYE SHADOW

ELECTRIC RED ORANGE LOOSE PIGMENT

PINKY CHAMPAGNE EYE SHADOW

DARK BROWN EYEBROW PENCIL

DARK BROWN EYEBROW SHADOW

EYE MAKEUP REMOVER

ORANGE PEACH CREAM BLUSH

BLACK GEL LINER

BLACK MASCARA

1 SET BIG PLUSH STRIP LASHES

DARK DUO

LIGHT PEACH LOOSE POWDER

SHIMMERY CORAL PEACH BLUSH

HOT PINK LIP LINER

HOT PINK LIP GLOSS

FOUNDATION BRUSHES

BEAUTYBLENDER

EYE SHADOW BRUSHES

ANGLED EYEBROW BRUSH

EYELINER BRUSH

EYELASH CURLER

SMALL FAN BRUSH

ORANGEWOOD STICK

POWDER BRUSH

BLUSH BRUSH

LIP BRUSH

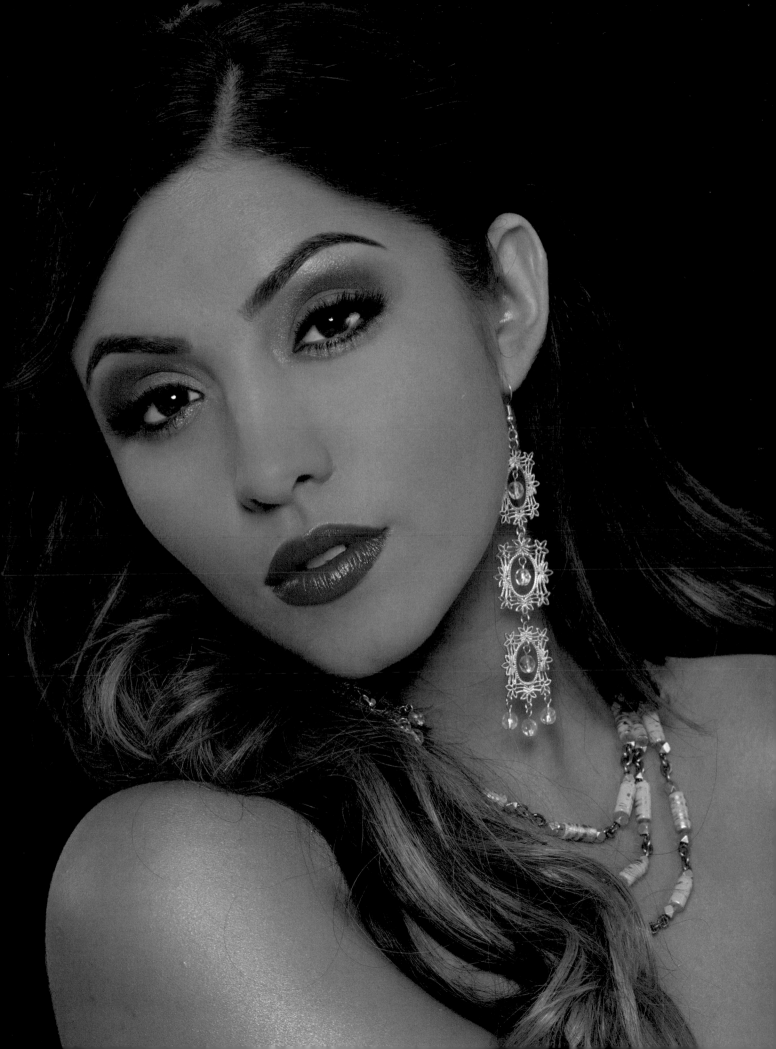

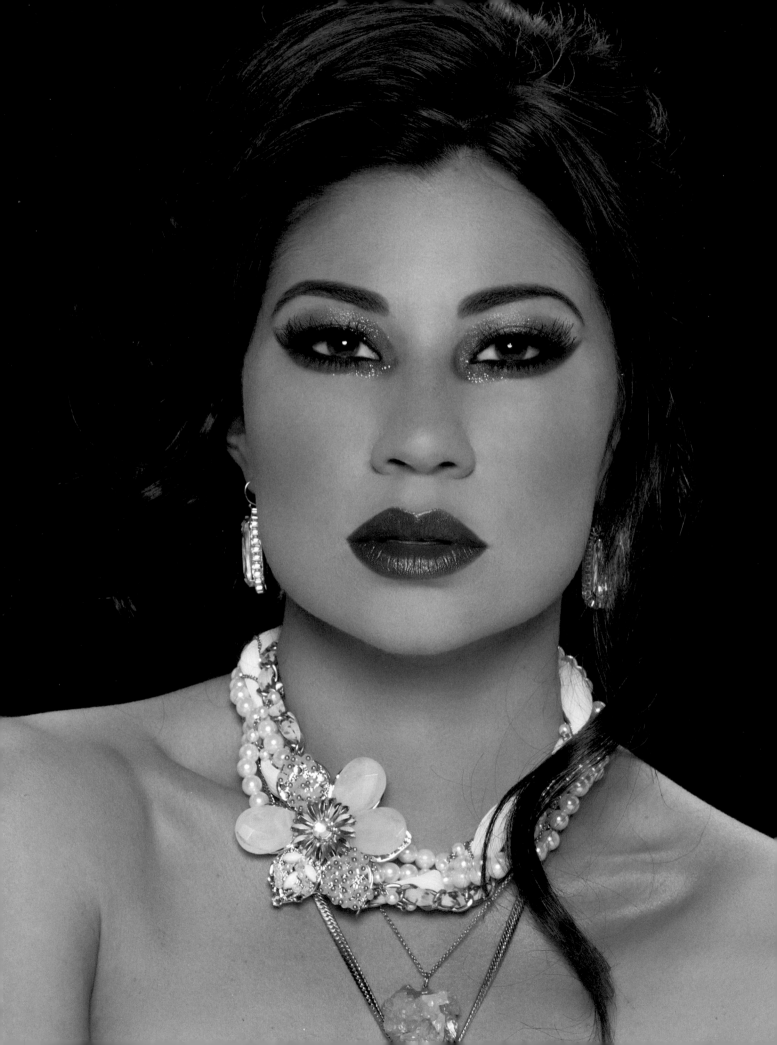

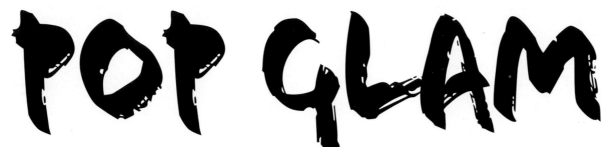

POP GLAM

When I was young and with friends getting ready to go out, we'd often blast music. Prince was one of our favorites. His early work inspired the brilliant purple/blue used on the lids in this image. For extra pop and sparkle, keep unexpected colors on hand like the fuchsia used here. Her eyes look like sparkling gems. This is fun party makeup and relatively easy to create.

* Apply foundation to the eyes and the forehead up into the hairline.

* Brush out the eyebrows.

* With a fluffy eyeliner brush, go under the eye with a bright red loose pigment. (Wet the tip of the brush and flare up and out for a more defined point.)

* Apply fluorescent pink loose pigment with a rounded eyeliner brush around the inner eye and tear duct, blending under the eye.

* Apply a bright violet blue eye shadow all over the lid and a little up to the outer crease. Keep blending in, and then, with a clean fluffy eye shadow brush, blend out the edges.

* Apply clear wax and dark brown eyebrow shadow with an angled eyebrow brush for a beautiful dramatic brow.

* Apply reflects pigment with a violet pink hue all over the lid to the brow and under the eye with a fluffy eye shadow brush.

* Clean up any excess with eye makeup remover.

* Curl the lashes and apply mascara.

* Line the inner upper and lower waterlines and line on top of the lash line in a nice cat line using black gel liner and a pointy eyeliner brush.

* Apply two sets of long Wispies strip lashes, one on top of the other, using dark Duo.

* Apply mascara again.

* Apply foundation to the rest of the face, neck, and ears.

* Apply a baby pink cream blush.

* Apply a ruby purple lipstick all over the lips. Top off the lips with a raspberry lip gloss. Blot.

* Apply a bright pink blush with a fluffy blush brush.

* Lightly dust the face with translucent powder.

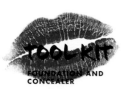

TOOLKIT

FOUNDATION AND CONCEALER

BRIGHT RED LOOSE PIGMENT

FLUORESCENT PINK LOOSE PIGMENT

BRIGHT VIOLET BLUE EYE SHADOW

CLEAR WAX AND DARK BROWN EYEBROW SHADOW

REFLECTS LOOSE PIGMENT WITH A VIOLET/PINK HUE

MAKEUP REMOVER

BLACK MASCARA

BLACK GEL LINER

2 SETS LONG WISPIES STRIP LASHES

DARK DUO

BABY PINK CREAM BLUSH

RUBY PURPLE LIPSTICK

RASPBERRY LIP GLOSS

BRIGHT PINK BLUSH

TRANSLUCENT POWDER

FOUNDATION BRUSHES

BEAUTYBLENDER

ANGLED EYEBROW BRUSH

EYELINER BRUSHES

EYE SHADOW BRUSHES

EYELASH CURLER

SMALL FAN BRUSH

ORANGEWOOD STICK

FLUFFY BLUSH BRUSH

POWDER BRUSH

LIP BRUSH

TRANQUIL

For this look, I wanted to create a sexy and glamorous blue eye. Dasia has great eyes that have lots of lid, a nice crease, and a beautiful brow bone. She also has wonderful bone structure with beautiful high Native American cheekbones. The blues and oranges remind me of when the blue waters at Laguna Beach hit the bright orange sunset. This is a fun look for hitting the dance floor.

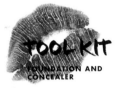

TOOL KIT

FOUNDATION AND CONCEALER

MIDNIGHT BLUE CREAM EYE SHADOW

SHIMMERY BRIGHT BLUE LOOSE PIGMENT

MINT GREEN CREAM EYE SHADOW

LAVENDER BLUE SHIMMERY LOOSE PIGMENT

BRIGHT ORANGE MATTE EYE SHADOW

CLEAR WAX AND DARK BROWN EYEBROW SHADOW

BLACK GEL LINER

BONE-COLORED EYELINER PENCIL

BLACK MASCARA

1 SET DEMI WISPIES STRIP LASHES

DARK DUO

INDIVIDUAL FLARE LASHES IN SHORT, MEDIUM, AND LONG

EYE MAKEUP REMOVER

SHEER CORAL CREAM BLUSH

TRANSLUCENT POWDER

RED BLUSH

DEEP RED LIP PENCIL

RED LIPSTICK

FOUNDATION BRUSHES

BEAUTYBLENDER

LIP BRUSHES

EYE SHADOW BRUSHES

EYELINER BRUSHES

ANGLED EYEBROW BRUSH

EYELASH CURLER

SMALL FAN BRUSH

ORANGEWOOD STICK

TWEEZERS

POWDER BRUSH

CONTOURED BLUSH BRUSH

✳ Apply foundation all over the eyes and up onto the forehead and into the hairline.

✳ With midnight blue cream eye shadow, paint a triangle with a lip brush from the center of the lid, diagonally up and out past the crease, then back down under the outer corner of the eye, and fill in.

✳ Apply a shimmery bright blue loose pigment over the triangle.

✳ Apply mint green cream eye shadow with a fat eyeliner brush along the bottom of the eye.

✳ With an eye shadow brush, apply a lavender blue shimmery loose pigment in a circular motion to the inner upper eyelid and up to the crease, and ever so slightly blend on top of the midnight blue for a nice fade.

✳ Apply the same lavender blue shimmery loose pigment on top of the mint green cream eye shadow under the eye; blend up to the outer corner of eye with an eye shadow brush.

✳ Apply a bright orange matte eye shadow above the upper outer crease of the eye, fading up toward the brow.

✳ With a small thin crease eye shadow brush, apply midnight blue cream eye shadow toward the crease. Blend well.

✳ Apply clear wax and dark brown eyebrow shadow with an angled eyebrow brush to sculpt the eyebrows into an intense outer arch.

✳ Line the upper lash line with black gel liner and a pointy eyeliner brush.

✳ Line the inner upper and lower waterlines with a bone-colored eyeliner pencil.

✳ Curl the lashes and apply mascara.

✳ Apply one set of Demi Wispies strip lashes with dark Duo. Lay individual flare lashes in short, medium, and long into the lash line.

✳ Line the upper lash line tightly with a black gel liner. Apply mascara again.

✳ Clean up under the eyes with makeup remover. Put some makeup remover on the edge of the sponge; press the corner of the sponge upward at the outer corner of the eye to sharpen the edge of the makeup.

✳ Apply foundation to the rest of the face, neck, and ears.

✳ Apply a sheer coral cream blush.

✳ Blend this all in with foundation brushes and a Beautyblender.

✳ Use a brush to dust the whole face with translucent powder.

✳ Apply red blush and lightly brush up toward the outer corner of the eye with a contoured blush brush.

✳ Line the lips with a deep red lip pencil and then top off the lips with a red lipstick.

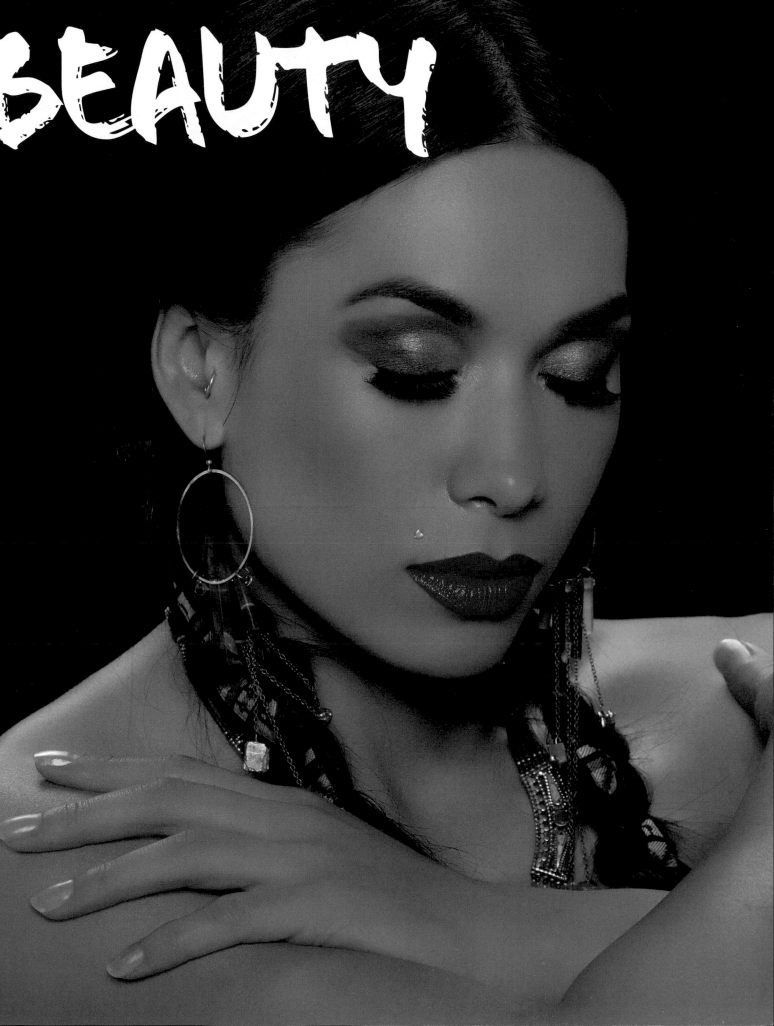

BEAUTY

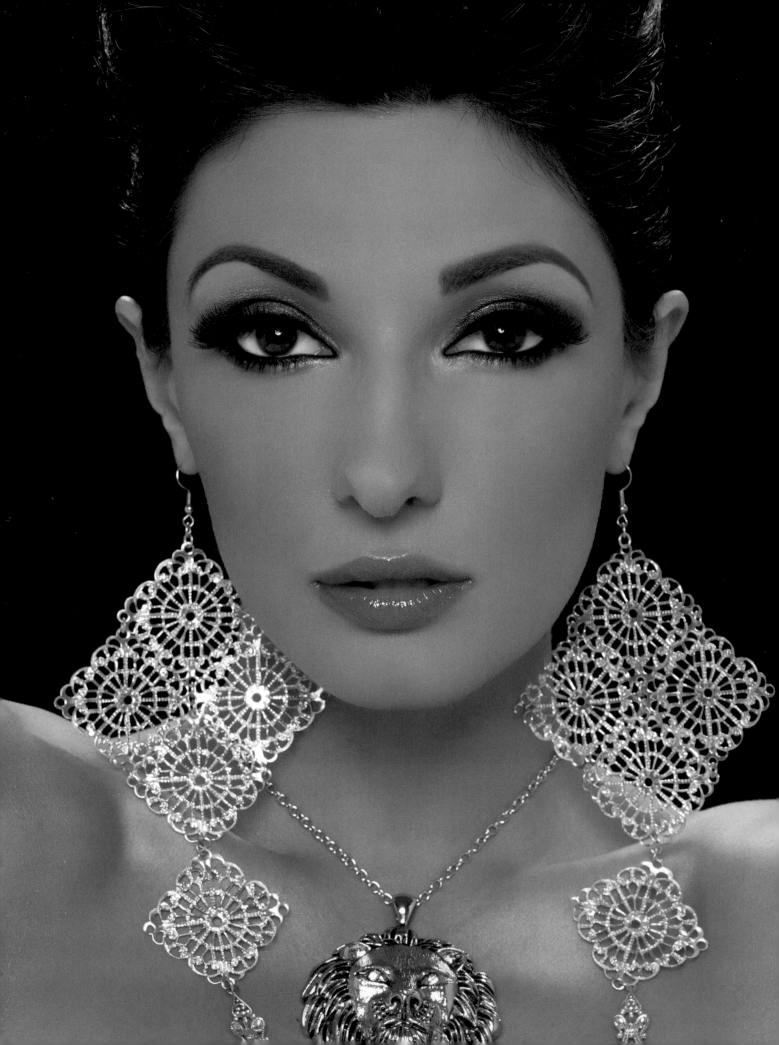

These rich and smoky eyes will lure in any prince or king out of the desert for well over 1,001 nights. I love mixing the bright color with gold and with the rich black. This look evokes hot, humid nights, nightclubs, and throbbing music.

* Apply foundation to the eyes and forehead and up into the hairline.

* With a brown eyebrow pencil, draw in the eyebrows, creating a curved arch, and then extend out the brow.

* Using an angled eyebrow brush, apply clear wax with brown eyebrow shadow and fill in on top of the pencil to soften the brows up a bit.

* Apply a royal blue cream eye shadow to the lids.

* With a small eye shadow brush, apply gold loose pigment to the inner eye, around the tear duct, and all under the eye.

* Apply a bright sparkly royal blue loose pigment on top of the blue cream eye shadow and blend well with a fluffy eye shadow brush.

* Apply black loose pigment with gold sparkles to the outer eye and under the corner of the eye, blending into the crease and onto the outer lid.

* Line the inner upper and lower waterlines and inner tear duct with black gel liner; line the upper lash line with a cat line.

* Curl the lashes and apply mascara.

* Apply two sets of plush strip lashes that are different from each other with dark Duo.

* Apply mascara again.

* Apply foundation to the rest of the face, neck, and ears.

* Mix a rose gold body makeup into foundation and apply all over the chest and upper cheekbones.

* Dab a light gold makeup under the lip in the middle of the chin.

* Apply a coral cream blush to the cheeks.

* Blend this all in with foundation brushes and a Beautyblender.

* Powder the face with translucent powder and a powder brush.

* Apply a peach blush to the cheekbones with a blush brush.

* Apply a sparkly sheer peach lip gloss.

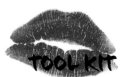

TOOL KIT

FOUNDATION AND CONCEALER

BROWN EYEBROW PENCIL

CLEAR WAX AND BROWN EYEBROW SHADOW

ROYAL BLUE CREAM EYE SHADOW

GOLD LOOSE PIGMENT

BRIGHT SPARKLY ROYAL BLUE LOOSE PIGMENT

BLACK LOOSE PIGMENT WITH GOLD SPARKLES

BLACK GEL LINER

BLACK MASCARA

2 SETS PLUSH STRIP LASHES, EACH DIFFERENT

DARK DUO

ROSE GOLD BODY MAKEUP

LIGHT GOLD MAKEUP

CORAL CREAM BLUSH

TRANSLUCENT POWDER

PEACH BLUSH

SPARKLY SHEER PEACH LIP GLOSS

FOUNDATION BRUSHES

BEAUTYBLENDER

ANGLED EYEBROW BRUSH

EYE SHADOW BRUSHES

EYELINER BRUSHES

EYELASH CURLER

SMALL FAN BRUSH

ORANGEWOOD STICK

POWDER BRUSH

BLUSH BRUSH

LIP BRUSH

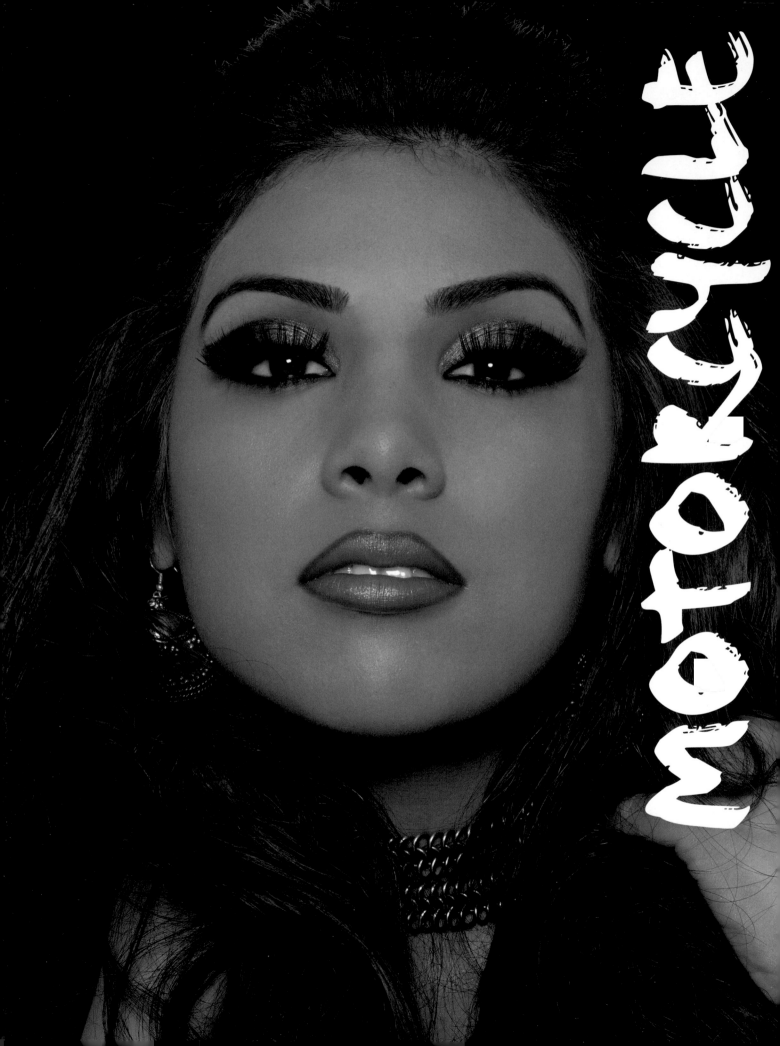

motorcycle

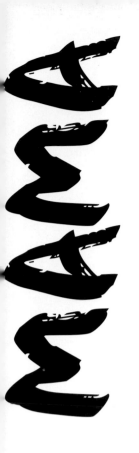

MAMA

Just because she is riding the back of a bike all over the country does not mean that she can't look incredibly sexy while looking tough at the same time. This look is about sculpted brows and fiercely sculpted almond eyes. Midnight blue eyes with kissable pink lips will not steer you wrong.

* Apply foundation to the eyes and forehead up into the hairline.

* With a dark brown eyebrow pencil, draw on top of the eyebrows to heighten and to really give a high arch that sweeps down dramatically.

* Using an angled eyebrow brush, fill in the brow thickly, using clear wax and a dark brown eyebrow shadow. Brush up the beginning of the eyebrow.

* Apply a bronzy peach eye shadow to the inner eye and blend in a circular motion up to under the brow and then all the way under the eye.

* Apply a bright blue cream eye shadow to the lids; at the inner eye, draw out above the outer crease in a defined rounded swoop with a bit of a very thick cat line.

* With a small eye shadow brush, apply a blue loose pigment on top of the cream eye shadow.

* Use a small eye shadow brush to apply a jet black cream eye shadow to the outer corners of the eye just from the middle of the eye. Blend in, but keep the line at the crease precise. With an eyeliner brush and black gel liner, draw a line to give even more precision at the crease.

* Line the inner upper and lower waterlines and inner tear duct with

black gel liner; line tightly under the eye as well.

* Curl the lashes and apply mascara.

* Apply two sets of strip lashes, one that is full and plush and one that is huge, spiky, and vampy, with dark Duo.

* Line the upper lash line with black gel liner again to help hide the lash bands.

* Apply mascara again.

* Clean up under the eyes with makeup remover.

* Apply foundation to the rest of the face, neck, and ears.

* Contour down the sides of the nose, just under the upper cheekbones, and under the jawline with a light brown cream contour color.

* Apply a brown nude cream blush.

* Blend this all in with foundation brushes and a Beautyblender.

* Powder the face with light peach loose powder and a powder puff, fluffing off any excess with a brush.

* Apply a mauve pink blush to the cheeks with an angled blush brush.

* Line the lips with a mauve brown lip pencil. Do not fill in.

* Apply a light pale pink lipstick to the lips.

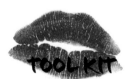

TOOL KIT

FOUNDATION AND CONCEALER

DARK BROWN EYEBROW PENCIL

CLEAR WAX AND DARK BROWN EYEBROW SHADOW

BRONZY PEACH EYE SHADOW

BRIGHT BLUE CREAM EYE SHADOW

BLUE LOOSE PIGMENT

JET BLACK CREAM EYE SHADOW

BLACK GEL LINER

BLACK MASCARA

1 SET PLUSH STRIP LASHES

1 SET SUPER BIG SPIKY VAMPY STRIP LASHES

DARK DUO

EYE MAKEUP REMOVER

LIGHT BROWN CREAM CONTOUR COLOR

BROWN NUDE CREAM BLUSH

LIGHT PEACH LOOSE POWDER

MAUVE PINK BLUSH

MAUVE BROWN LIP PENCIL

LIGHT PALE PINK LIPSTICK

FOUNDATION BRUSHES

BEAUTYBLENDER

ANGLED EYEBROW BRUSH

EYEBROW COMB

EYE SHADOW BRUSHES

EYELINER BRUSHES

EYELASH CURLER

SMALL FAN BRUSH

ORANGEWOOD STICK

POWDER PUFF

POWDER BRUSH

ANGLED BLUSH BRUSH

LIP BRUSH

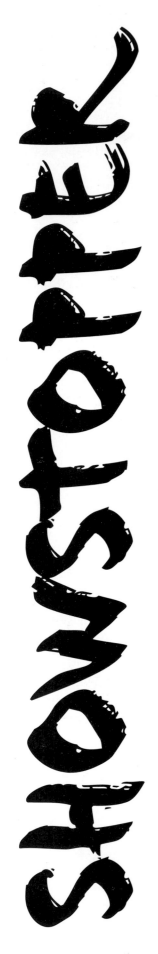

Kiersy is a beautiful, sweet young woman, and I try to book her whenever possible. She told me this was the first time getting that glammed up and she loved it. With this series, I went for eighties couture with a strong influence of punk. This is glamorous and sexy. The color scheme is worn brass, copper, silver, gold, and black.

✳ Apply foundation to over the eyes, up over the eyebrow, and into the forehead and hairline.

✳ Apply a rusty brown eye shadow all over the eyelid up to the crease, close to the tear duct, and then above the crease line toward the outer eye.

✳ Apply matte silver loose pigment with a regular small eye shadow brush above the top tear duct onto the inner lid.

✳ Apply matte gold loose pigment to the outer lid and eye up to the brow.

✳ Apply matte bronze loose pigment to the upper crease and down around the outer eye.

✳ Apply rich chocolate brown loose pigment to the outer lid up to the crease.

✳ With a clean eye shadow brush, blend the edges of all colors into one another.

✳ The next steps use black gel liner and eyeliner brushes.

✳ Line all the way under the eye and off toward the temple.

✳ Line the upper lash line from the tear duct and out in a thick cat line, connecting with a point under the eye.

✳ Line the tear duct and point toward the nose; using that as your starting point for the crease line, line up the inner eye and over the crease, dramatically trailing off the eye.

✳ Line the inner upper and lower waterlines and inner tear duct.

✳ Line on top of the eyebrows with a thin brush to create real definition.

✳ With an angled eyebrow brush, apply a little brown eyebrow shadow to the brows at the beginning, fading to the arch.

✳ Use a fluffy eyeliner brush and a matte black eye shadow to buff the crease, but don't soften too much.

✳ Curl the lashes and apply mascara with a mascara wand.

✳ Remove fallen makeup from under the eye with makeup remover.

✳ Apply black individual flare lashes in short, medium, and long, layering each for full coverage, with dark Duo.

✳ Apply one set of plush strip lashes with dark Duo.

✳ Apply one set of Wispies strip lashes with dark Duo.

✳ Apply matte silver loose pigment just under the center of the eye.

✳ Apply mascara again.

✳ Apply foundation to the rest of the face.

✳ Contour the jawline with a brown cream contour color.

✳ Apply a light yellow gold makeup to the upper cheeks, below the lip, and above the eyebrow.

✳ Blend this all in with foundation brushes and a Beautyblender.

✳ Fill in the entire lip with black gel liner.

✳ Apply matte gold loose pigment on the lips.

✳ Top off the lips with a clear lip gloss.

✳ Lightly dust the face with translucent powder.

✳ Apply a bronze gold body makeup all over the body.

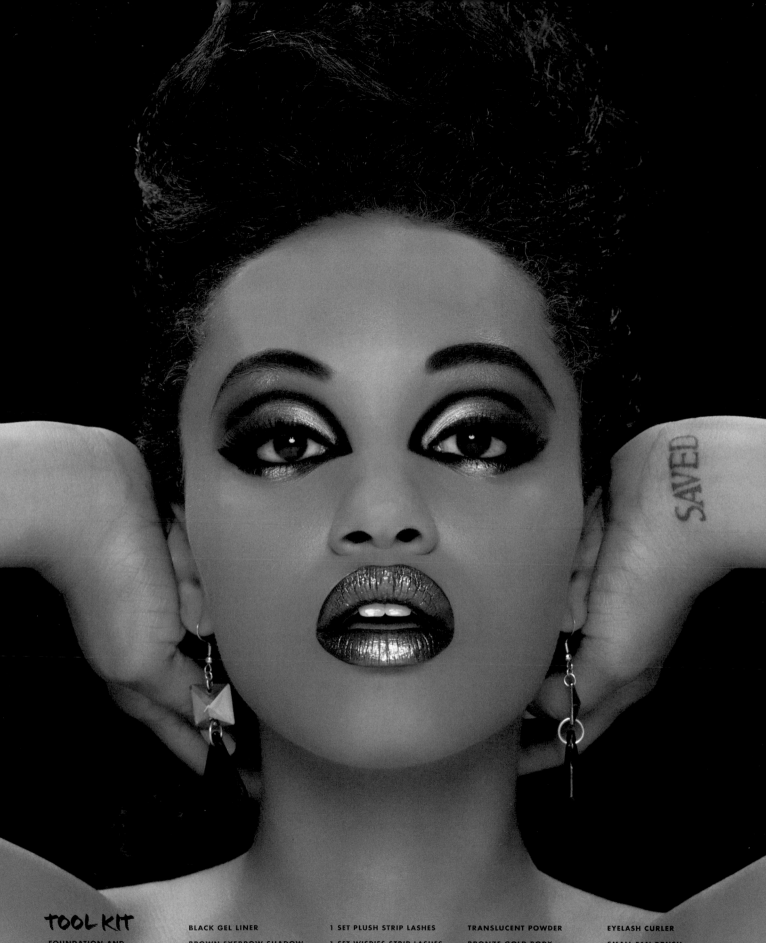

TOOL KIT

FOUNDATION AND
CONCEALER

RUSTY BROWN EYE
SHADOW

MATTE SILVER, GOLD, AND
BRONZE LOOSE PIGMENTS

RICH CHOCOLATE BROWN
LOOSE PIGMENT

BLACK GEL LINER

BROWN EYEBROW SHADOW

MATTE BLACK EYE SHADOW

BLACK MASCARA

EYE MAKEUP REMOVER

BLACK INDIVIDUAL FLARE
LASHES IN SHORT, MEDIUM,
AND LONG

1 SET PLUSH STRIP LASHES

1 SET WISPIES STRIP LASHES

DARK DUO

BROWN CREAM CONTOUR
COLOR

LIGHT YELLOW GOLD
MAKEUP

CLEAR LIP GLOSS

TRANSLUCENT POWDER

BRONZE GOLD BODY
MAKEUP

FOUNDATION BRUSHES

BEAUTYBLENDER

EYE SHADOW BRUSHES

EYELINER BRUSHES

ANGLED EYEBROW BRUSH

EYELASH CURLER

SMALL FAN BRUSH

MASCARA WAND

TWEEZERS

ORANGEWOOD STICK

POINTY LIP BRUSH

REGULAR LIP BRUSH

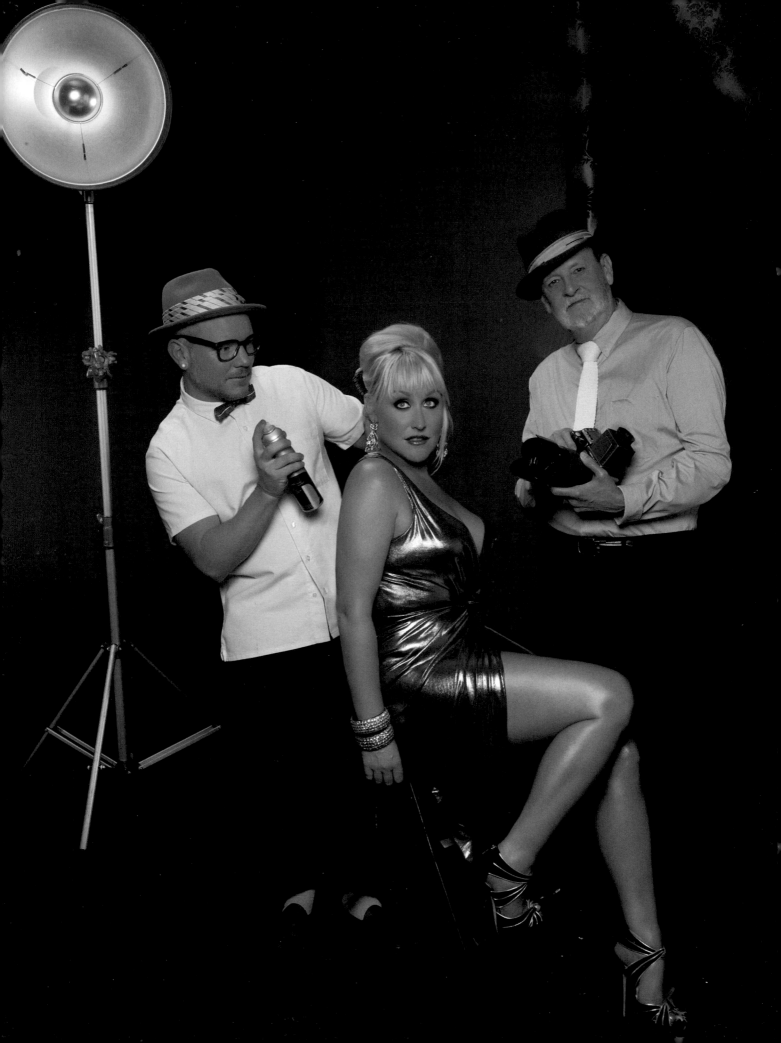

ACKNOWLEDGMENTS

This book was such a labor of love, not only for me but for everyone involved. I have never experienced anything in my career that can compare. This is a dream come true! I must first and foremost thank Kevyn Aucoin, the brilliant makeup artist who lit the makeup fire within me; I still refer to his books to this day and they are the reason I wanted to have a book of my own. I am also very grateful and inspired by the photographer David LaChapelle; I cherish his books and images. Both of these gentlemen have heavily influenced me and this book. I could not have done this without my family's constant support. My great-grandma Nana, Sunny Thomas; my grandma Pat Felix (Glamma); and my mom, Suni Johnson, are the reason I am who I am, and I am forever grateful. I also must mention the rest of my family who mean so much to me—your unending support and love is never unnoticed! My brother, Taylor Johnson, and his wife, Susan Johnson; my cousin, Nick Felix, and his wife, Pauline Felix; my Big Daddy Joe Felix; David Hostetter; my uncle John Felix and my aunt Donna Carroll; Stephen Johnson; and my dad, John Mills. And of course my loving daughter, Solaris.

I am fortunate to have many true friends in my life who always encourage me and help ease my worries and push me to move forward. Not only do we have way too much fun, but you have also stood by me through thick and thin. Special thanks to my girls Amber Gayner, Nancy Stimac, Chanda Hutton, Fiona Locke, Nadege Shoenfeld, Jana DeGrange, Lori Bursik, and Joanna Nelson. Michael Johnston and Patti Brand-Reese—man, did you guys get me through the last three years! I love our friendship and our working relationship; your support meant more than you realize—oh, the things we have been through!

David Alley, we did it! What an amazing roller coaster ride this was. Thank you for believing in me and in this amazing project. Your photography is, as everyone can see, off the hook! Thank you, thank you, thank you! Ivette Chornomud: Thank you for all the photo retouching and compositing. I cannot thank both of you enough for working with the pressure of the deadlines; we made 'em!

Huge thanks to all of the beautiful faces that inspired me and joined me on this ride. Thank you for letting me play. There is nothing like a muse!

I must also thank John O'Mally, for helping me make sense of this book, and Susan Hashimoto, for helping me put the first original photographs and ideas together in a proposal. John, not only did you help put the proposal and book together, but you also helped me complete it—thank you! Of course, Mom, thank you for your input and help with the writing and editing. Nick Greenbury, you were by my side on all of the long days of the prep, shoot, and post, and thank you for your support and help with the writing, rewriting, and editing. April Neale, for standing by through all the highs and lows and then introducing me to Jeff Silberman. Jeff, for looking out for me and getting it into the right hands and then guiding me through it all. Of course Penguin and Jeanette Shaw, for believing in my vision and making this dream a reality. Aubrey Loots, I feel blessed to have you in my life and as one of my best friends. You are such an incredible inspiration and really are definitely one of the best hair dressers I know! Thank you and your Studio DNA team with special thanks to: Jonathan Mason, Jamie Pierce, and Dane Tuttle—the hair in this book looks beyond amazing. Tiffany Hughes, my makeup assistant, standing by my side and constantly organizing me: I could not have done it without your backbreaking help! More than anything, with both the hair and makeup teams, it is our friendship—your great vibes and major support is what bleeds through onto these pages. Thank you to Audrey Brianne and her assistant, Tara Hunt, for the wardrobe and jewelry styling—you guys are amazing! All the fab designers who came to the table: thank you, Curly Vee, David Profeta, Valerej Propeja, and Summer Rose—your designs helped add to the uniqueness of this book. Thank you, Kitten Hawk, Kuumba Vanessa Mooney, Evil Pawn Jewelry, American Apparel, Venice Vintage Paradise, Albertus Swanepoel, Britt by Britt, Dogeared, Natalie B. Designs, Jenny Dayco, and CAROLEE.

Thank you, David Tayar and Jeanne Tyson, for your presence and documenting it all; Jason Barajas, for the props and set dressing designs; the lighting, grip, and camera tech team: Frank Shaffer, Cameron Wong, and John Shin; Kirk Huston and your amazing 1971 Ford Bronco; Mad Dog Studios; and SkyThrills and the beautiful yellow plane!

Last but not least, thank you to my Gleam Team! Gleam would not even exist without the support, help, and love that my grandma Pat Felix and mom Suni Johnson have poured in. Lindsey Teel and Joanna Nelson, Gleam Team extraordinaires, your hard work never goes unnoticed. Last but not least, thank you Matt Walker and Olivia Salta Formaggio with Period Media, Thank you!

Special thanks to Nicholous Greenbury. You were my rock through all of this. You stood by my side 24/7, kept me positive, and helped to align my thoughts. Your love is beyond anything I have experienced, and I am so happy to have had each other to experience this amazing ride. Here's to another one . . .

CREDITS

All photography by David Alley.
All hair styling by Aubrey Loots of Studio DNA unless otherwise noted.
All wardrobe and jewelry styling by Audrey Brianne unless otherwise noted.

Page ii: Hair by Kimi Messina; wardrobe styling by David Profeta

Page 2: Hair by Kimi Messina; wardrobe styling by David Profeta

Page 16: Skin finishing by Fiona Locke

Page 19: Hair by Kimi Messina; makeup by Patti Ramsey-Bortoli

Page 21: Costume design by Curly V

Page 23: Photo compositing by Ivette G. Chornomud

Pages 55: Photo compositing by David Alley

Page 56: Hair by Kimi Messina; wardrobe styling by Summer Rose

Page 58: Dress by Tatyana Peter; wardrobe styling by Summer Rose

Pages 60, 61: Hair by Kimi Messina

Page 63: Wardrobe styling by Summer Rose; hair by Dane Tuttle

Page 64: Hair by Cynthia Romo and Nancy Stimac; wardrobe styling by Summer Rose

Page 67: Hair by Kimi Messina; wardrobe styling by David Profeta

Page 68: Costume design by Summer Rose

Page 71: Costume design by Summer Rose

Page 74: Costume design by Summer Rose

Page 77: Cape designed by Valerj Probega

Page 79: Body painting by Tyson Fontaine

Page 80: Costume design by Summer Rose

Page 83: Photo compositing by Ivette G. Chornomud

Page 84: Hair by Kimi Messina

Page 87: Costume design by Curly V

Page 91: Hair by Kimi Messina

Page 92: Costume design by Summer Rose

Page 96: Hair by Dane Tuttle; wardrobe styling by Summer Rose

Page 99: Hair by Nancy Stimic; wardrobe styling by Summer Rose

Page 100: Costume design by Curly V

Page 103: Hair by Kimi Messina; costume design by Randall Christensen

Page 104: Hair by Kimi Messina

Page 106: Photo compositing by Ivette G. Chornomud

Page 146: Makeup by Brigitta Hennech

Page 149: Makeup by Brigitta Hennech

ABOUT THE AUTHOR

Emmy Award–winning makeup artist **Melanie Mills** is one of Hollywood's leading style-makers and beauty consultants, known for her glamorous flair, supreme talent, and vivacious personality. Melanie's journey began in Thousand Oaks, California, but she soon ventured throughout the world, living, learning, and making memories that would leave lifelong impressions not only on her but on those she encountered. Born to a family of intelligent, strong, and capable women, each style icons in their own right, Melanie's love affair with glitter, glam, and all things stylish was her true destiny.

Today, Melanie is one of the most sought-after makeup experts in the industry. With more than fourteen years of experience, Melanie is a master of her craft, sculpting faces and bodies to true works of art in a variety of mediums, including television, film, and editorial.

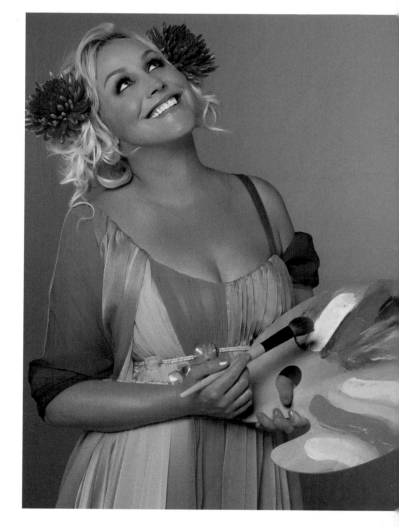

In 2007, Melanie was selected as the Makeup Department Head for ABC television's global phenomenon *Dancing with the Stars*, where she redefined the look of the series and won the Emmy Award for Outstanding Makeup Design in 2008. Melanie's superior talent has earned her nine career Emmy nominations for her work on various projects in the entertainment industry, including two double nominations.

While working with *Dancing with the Stars*, Melanie created Gleam Body Radiance, a revolutionary new transfer-resistant body makeup that perfects and illuminates the skin in four shades and is sold worldwide (www.gleambymelaniemills.com). Expanding her beauty collection, Melanie launched Gleam Lip Radiance in February 2012, made with organic and botanical ingredients that lasts all day or all night long. Melanie continues to expand Gleam by Melanie Mills with new and exciting products, many of which are featured in this book. Melanie's products and tips for creating flawless makeup for the face and body have appeared on *The Dr. Oz Show*, *The Talk*, *Home and Family*, and *Access Hollywood Live* and in national publications, including *Allure*, *Shape*, *Vogue*, *InStyle*, *US Weekly*, *OK*, *Redbook*, *Emmy*, *Essence*, and *People*, among others.

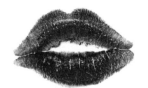